WITHDRAWN

The Psychobiology of Chronic Headache

Donald A. Bakal, Ph.D., is Director of the Headache Research Project at the University of Calgary and is also Professor of Psychology in the University of Calgary Department of Psychology and the University of Calgary Medical School Division of Psychiatry. He received his doctorate in psychology in 1971 from the University of Manitoba. His theoretical and empirical writings are recognized by clinicians and researchers throughout the world.

The Psychobiology of Chronic Headache

Donald A. Bakal, Ph.D.

 Springer Publishing Company
New York

To Janice

Copyright © 1982 by Springer Publishing Company, Inc.

All rights reserved.

No part of this publication may be reproduced, stored in a retrieval system, or transmitted in any form or by any means, electronic, mechanical, photocopying, recording, or otherwise, without the prior permission of Springer Publishing Company, Inc.

Springer Publishing Company, Inc.
200 Park Avenue South
New York, New York 10003

82 83 84 85 86/10 9 8 7 6 5 4 3 2 1

Library of Congress Cataloging in Publication Data

Bakal, Donald A.
  The psychobiology of chronic headache.

  Bibliography: p.
  Includes index.
  1. Headache—Psychological aspects. 2. Headache—Psychosomatic aspects. 3. Chronic diseases—Psychological aspects. I. Title. [DNLM: 1. Headache. WL 342 B166p]
RC392.B335 1982   616.8'49   82-10363
ISBN 0-8261-3890-X

Printed in the United States of America

Contents

Preface	vii
1. The Psychobiological Model	1
2. Stress Versus Distress	10
Coping Styles and Headache Susceptibility	18
3. Physiological Mechanisms	27
Vascular Mechanisms	28
Musculoskeletal Activity and Headache Susceptibility	33
Cerebral Blood Flow Studies	38
Instability of the Autonomic Nervous System	42
The Origin of Pain	44
4. One or More Kinds of Headache?	48
Classification of Headache	50
Empirical Observations of Headache Symptoms	55
Headache Symptoms in Children	65
Headache Symptoms in the Population	70
5. Clinical and Theoretical Concerns	77
Dimension Versus Syndrome	77
The Role of Drugs in Headache Management	81
What of Physical Triggers?	92
6. Behavioral Approaches to Treatment	100
Biofeedback	100
Cognitive Skills Training	109
Summary	118

7. **A Manual for the Cognitive Behavioral Treatment of Chronic Headache**   120
   The Patient's Conceptualization of Headache   123
   Relaxation/Biofeedback Training   126
   Attention-Diversion Training   138
   Imagery Training   141
   Thought Management   145

Conclusion   148

References   151

Index   161

Preface

The content of this book represents a new approach to understanding headache sufferers and their symptoms. The approach evolved during eight years of research and clinical interactions with chronic headache patients and represents a collective effort involving myself and my colleagues Judith Ann Kaganov and Stefan Demjen. We also were influenced heavily in our thinking by the many headache sufferers who attended our clinic over the years and who shared their insights concerning the courses and management of chronic headache disorders.

The need for a new understanding of headache sufferers is not difficult to document. It has been said that chronic headache competes with the common cold as the most common health problem. Moreover, headache is one of the most frequent reasons for individuals seeking medical treatments, and it accounts for an astronomical number of office visits to family practitioners, neurologists, pediatricians, and surgical specialists. It is almost paradoxical that headache is such a large problem to a society that has the most advanced health-care system in the world. The situation might be considered even humorous were it not for the pain, misery, and suffering of those afflicted. I am not referring here to individuals who can control "everyday" headache with an aspirin or two but rather to those unfortunate individuals who experience severe headache attacks on a daily or near-daily basis. Many of these individuals have been in this condition for a large portion of their adolescent and adult lives. Medications are no longer effective for these individuals and their only relief comes with sleep. However, sleep is accompanied by the realization that upon awakening the pain and suffering will most likely be present once again.

Most chronic headache sufferers realize that they will not die from headache, but at times they probably wish they would. The pain and suffering experienced by these individuals might be more bearable if they had a basis for understanding their affliction. They all have seen numerous physicians, neurological specialists, and even psychiatrists, but the outcome is generally the same. No cause for the disorder is found. Usually they are told to go home and "learn to live with the problem," but unfortunately no one tells them how. Many headache sufferers become so frustrated at being bounced from one specialist to another that they begin to hope that something physical will be found—even a tumor if it means that their suffering will be terminated.

Given this situation, it is not surprising to find headache sufferers constantly looking for the latest "cure" for their condition. Popular magazine articles, usually written by headache experts, advise readers to monitor their eating habits; to follow anti-headache diets; to use ion generators; or to try biofeedback, acupuncture, or hypnosis. Sometimes the religious adoption of one of these procedures may be accompanied by temporary relief, but usually the pain returns. I have seen many headache sufferers who at one time or another in their headache history obtained temporary relief from chiropractic exercises, diet, self-hypnosis, acupuncture, biofeedback, physiotherapy, or psychotherapy only to see their disorder return to its pretreatment level.

It is my thesis that a true understanding of the conditions controlling chronic headache can come only with the adoption of a holistic approach to the study of patients and their symptoms. Although the phrase *holistic approach* is very fashionable in academic circles at the moment, there is at the same time a poor understanding of what is meant by the phrase. For example, in some respects headache researchers have always been the exemplars of holistic medicine. For years, the medical founders of the American Association for the Study of Headache have encouraged colleagues from different disciplines to participate in their organization. And yet, there is still no clear sign that the research findings from one discipline (e.g., prostaglandin levels from biochemistry) have anything to do with the research findings from another discipline (e.g., MMPI profiles from psychology). The problem is that researchers from different disciplines do not have a common conceptual framework that allows them not just to share but to focus their empirical and clinical efforts on understanding headache patients and their symptoms.

It is necessary to emphasize that adopting a holistic approach to

Preface

the study of headache in no way precludes the collection of logical and physiological data in isolation from one another. However, it does require that researchers begin considering the manner in which their particular findings are related to the greater holistic or psychobiological condition of the headache sufferer. To give an example, several studies have demonstrated recently that cerebral blood flow changes during the painful state of a severe headache attack. None of these studies have considered the possibility that the observed vascular changes may be intricately related to the psychological state of the patient during the recording session. The position taken here is that the relationship between cerebral blood flow and experienced pain is bidirectional in that one cannot be understood without the other. Researchers can no longer proceed as if the physiological and psychological dimensions of human functioning operate independently from one another.

In this book, it is proposed that the holistic nature of chronic headache is best understood from a psychobiological perspective. At the heart of this approach is the assumption that the processes controlling the most common forms of chronic headache, muscle-contraction and migraine, are more similar than dissimilar. The approach challenges the almost universally held assumption that muscle-contraction and migraine headaches are different disorders with different etiologies and different symptoms, each requiring different forms of treatment. Traditional headache specialists describe muscle-contraction, or tension, headache as being characterized by sensations of tightness and persistent pain located in the neck and/or forehead regions. The pain is believed to result from sustained contraction of the head and neck muscles. On the other hand, migraine is described as a throbbing pain that is usually unilateral in nature and often associated with nausea, vomiting, and sensory disturbances prior to and during the actual headache attack. Migraine pain is believed to result from complex changes that take place in the cranial vasculature. In challenging the traditional muscle-contraction–migraine dichotomy, I do not wish to imply that one headache is the same as the next headache, for there are tremendous differences among individuals in terms of the head pain characteristics that they experience. Also, the same individuals often experience vastly different symptoms across attacks and even during attacks. The error has been in assuming that these between- and within-patient symptom differences are indicative of different disorders requiring different kinds of treatment. Moreover, a number of patient symptom similarities also exist, and the similarities may have stronger implications for understanding the etiology and treatment of chronic headache than do the differences.

In this context, one is reminded of the beginnings of Hans Selye's (1956) discovery of the *general adaptation syndrome*. In the introduction to his book *The Stress of Life*, Selye recalled that as a young medical student he was often more impressed by the similarities of patients with different physical symptoms than by the symptom features that were unique to each patient. He was intrigued by the fact that medical patients with a variety of infectious diseases all complained of similar diffuse aches and pains, or in his words were "all just plain sick." He recognized that this insight was not likely to endear him in the eyes of his superiors, so he decided not to pursue the idea until he had received his medical degree. Upon graduating, however, Selye began providing the scientific community with evidence to support his conviction that nonspecific factors are often as important as specific factors in understanding the origins of illness. He accomplished his objective without insisting that research into the specific factors of illness be altered. In a similar fashion, I hope to convince the reader that the understanding of headache can be enhanced by integrating psychological variables within knowledge of physiochemical processes that are believed to regulate the various symptom configurations seen in chronic headache sufferers.

The terms *psychobiological approach* and *severity approach* are used somewhat interchangeably throughout the text but at the same time with a slight difference in emphasis. Psychobiological is intended to convey the notion that a patient's susceptibility to headache, as well as the pain experienced during headache episodes, is a continuous and multifaceted condition involving cognitive, behavioral, physiological, and biochemical events. On the other hand, severity refers primarily to the notion that headache susceptibility and the symptoms experienced during headache attacks represent progressive conditions and that differences among headache sufferers can be understood in quantitative rather than qualitative terms.

The discussion begins with a chapter that outlines the psychobiological or severity model of headache followed by a chapter that deals with the physiological mechanisms believed to be involved in muscle-contraction and migraine headaches. As will be shown, there is considerable evidence that the physiological mechanisms controlling chronic headache operate along a continuum of severity. The next chapter deals with the symptom configurations commonly used to diagnose muscle-contraction and migraine headaches, along with the symptom configurations that are actually experienced by headache sufferers in clinical settings and in the general population. The physiological and symptom chapters are followed by a discussion of theoretical and clinical implications that the severity model has for physicians who are more accustomed to the traditional biomedical model of headache. The final two chapters deal with the treatment of headache, beginning with an overview of self-control methods of treatment and concluding with a detailed description of a structured cognitive behavioral headache management program.

The material that follows is presented with a mixture of excitement, conviction, and trepidation. A satisfactory understanding of headache patients and their symptoms has defied solution for hundreds of years, and for this reason alone a span of eight years may seem a dubious period for the incubation of a proper headache treatise. However, I believe that we have acquired sufficient knowledge, understanding, and data with which to proceed. In the final analysis, the utility of any new approach is determined not so much by its proponents as it is by those towards whom the approach is directed. Thus, the responses of clinicians, researchers, and headache sufferers themselves will in time determine the correctness of the decision to proceed.

1
The Psychobiological Model

Chronic headache sufferers and their symptoms need to be understood from a new perspective that integrates the various aspects of human functioning into one framework. What is needed is a conceptual model that explains the psychobiological processes that operate over-and-above the various psychological, social, physiological, and biochemical dimensions of human functioning. This model will help avoid the dualism inherent in our language that prevents our understanding of how different variables interact to produce headaches.

The conceptual shift that is required was well illustrated in an analogy first used by Frankl (1969). Frankl compared the human condition to that of a cylinder with a three-dimensional space (Figure 1.1). If the cylinder is projected out of its own three-dimensional space into lower horizontal and vertical dimensions, the result is two new dimensions with *different* properties. In one case the outcome is a circle; in the other case the outcome is a rectangle. In both cases something is lost, since the cylinder can never be fully understood in terms of the properties of the circle or the rectangle. If a human being is analyzed from a purely psychological or physiochemical frame of reference, the same limitations occur. In one case the outcome is psychological data; in the other case the outcome is biological data. In both cases the holistic perspective is lost. The cylinder analogy provides a convincing illustration of the distortions inherent in studying separate functions of persons rather than integrated living humans.

How can the cylinder analogy assist in the understanding of the chronic headache patient? Any patient who has undergone repeated

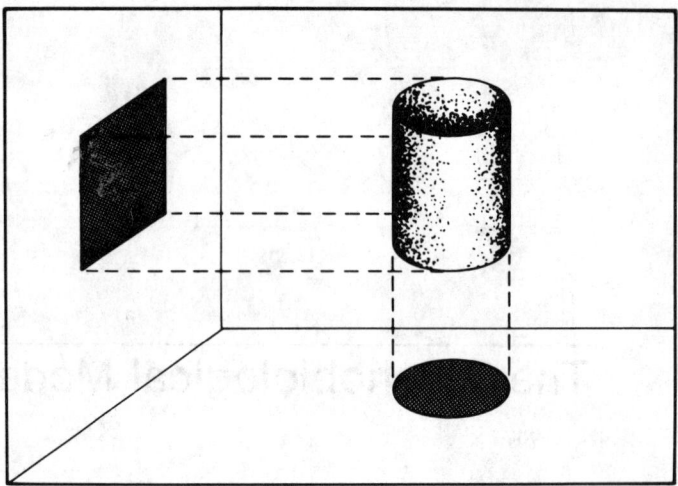

Figure 1.1 Projection of cylinder out of its three-dimensional space to form a circle and a rectangle; in both cases, something is lost (Frankl, 1969). Reprinted by permission of Hutchinson Publishing Group Limited.

medical examinations for recurring headache attacks knows that diagnostic and treatment techniques are based completely on the premise that the disorder must have either a psychological cause or a physical cause. Initially, the disorder may have been diagnosed as resulting from tension or stress, and the physician may have prescribed a muscle relaxant or a mild analgesic drug. If the problem persisted, the patient may have been advised to undergo a neurological examination. In many instances, neurological tests are necessary because there is always the possibility, no matter how remote, that a persistent headache complaint is indicative of some organic problem, such as a brain tumor. Almost invariably, however, a physical cause is not found. In the end, the patient may be given a new prescription for a more powerful drug; in some instances, the patient may even be referred to a psychiatrist. The following letter, which I received from a headache patient, is very characteristic of the plight facing these individuals:

> I have had migraine headaches for over five years... during this period I have received a number of neurological tests to rule out tumors, blockages, etc. All of the tests were negative and I was told that nothing was wrong with me physically. I have also seen a number of psychiatrists who have all told me that I had come to the wrong place and that they could do nothing to help me.

Observe that there was nothing physically or psychologically wrong with the patient. This dilemma characterizes virtually every person who suffers from chronic headache, and the dilemma will not be resolved until both professionals and patients recognize that headache is a condition involving the whole person. In discussing chronic pain, Sternbach (1974) has said that we should not speak of pain per se but rather only of pain patients. Exactly the same point is being made here. Recurring headache is the result of a multitude of variables that, taken together, make up the chronic headache sufferer.

A similar dualistic dilemma characterizes the research situation. Scientific meetings dealing with the causes and treatment of chronic headaches are generally attended by both medical and behavioral scientists, but the participants do not have a common conceptual framework for sharing their findings. In the morning sessions, medical researchers present and debate the latest biochemical findings, while the afternoon sessions are taken over by the behavioral scientists. Unfortunately, no forum exists for integrating the findings of one discipline with the findings of the other. It is quite possible that the findings of both disciplines are irrelevant to the problem at hand, which is understanding the headache patient in his/her entirety.

There is no magical solution to developing a holistic understanding of headache sufferers and their symptoms. However, as a first step towards a solution, I have proposed that the various aspects or dimensions of headache be considered within the context of a psychobiological model. As depicted in Figure 1.2, the model views chronic headache as resulting from complex transactions between environmental, psychological, physiological, genetic, and biochemical variables. The word *transaction* was deliberately chosen instead of the word *interaction* to connote a special kind of interplay that exists among the various components of the model. Lazarus (1978) first used the term *transactional process* to emphasize that in understanding stress reactions the relationship between environmental and person variables must be viewed as a two-way process, with both variables having mutual influence. Similarily, in the present context, *transaction* is meant to imply that the relationship between psychological and physiological components, as with the other components, is bidirectional in nature. Not only do psychological events influence physiological events, but physiological events also influence psychological events.

Transaction is also used in the present model with full awareness of Lazarus' belief that the study of human functioning must become more process-oriented. In fact, the emphasis of the psycho-

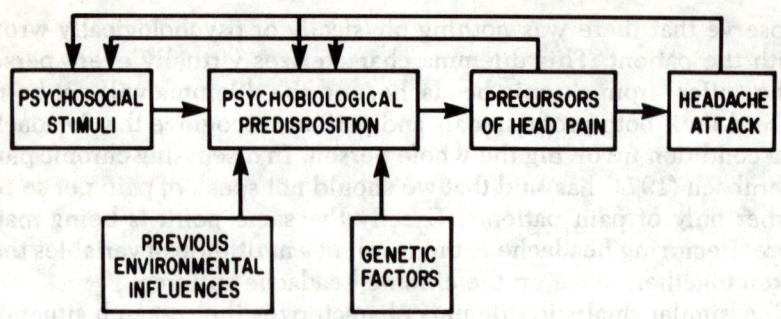

Figure 1.2 The psychobiological model of headache.

biological approach is not on what happened to these individuals in the past, either genetically or psychologically, but on what is happening to them now—during and across their uncontrollable attacks of pain. The past may be important for understanding the development of the disorder, but it has little significance for understanding the conditions that maintain the disorder. The word *transaction* also connotes the presence of emergent properties that cannot be identified from the separate study of the dimensions making up the model, or, as viewed by the Gestaltists, that the whole is more than the sum of its parts. In Lazarus' words, transaction implies a fusion of the components into a unit, a system, or a person.

In a similar fashion, Schwartz (1980) argued that the understanding of psychobiological disorders can be enhanced by moving away from an approach that looks for a single cause and towards an approach that incorporates the philosophy of general systems theory:

> ... at the most rudimentary level, general systems theory is concerned with the *behavior of any system* (atomic, chemical, cellular, organ, organism, social) ... The deep principle underlying systems theory, the one often missed or erroneously viewed as being trivial, is that the *behavior of a system emerges from dynamic interaction of its parts*. To understand how the system (any system) works as a *whole*, it becomes necessary to study its properties (its behavior) as a whole. This requires that the investigator appreciate the fact that complex and often unique *interactions* can occur between parts in a system. The parts, in interaction, are ultimately responsible for the unique properties or behaviors that occur when the system behaves as a whole. The concept of the "whole being greater than the sum of its parts but dependent upon the organization of the parts for its emergent properties as a whole" is at the heart of this realization. (p. 551)

The Psychobiological Model

There is one key component in the psychobiological model of headache that is roughly equivalent to the person or to the headache sufferer in his or her entirety. This component is called the *psychobiological predisposition,* and it represents a most crucial characteristic of chronic headache sufferers. Although partly initiated by genetic factors, its continued operation in the chronic headache patient goes well beyond genetic variables per se. The predisposition is seen as being a dynamic entity that is responsible for the increasing severity and chronicity of the headache patient's condition. During a particular attack, the predisposition is responsible for initiating the biochemical changes involved in the pain experience. In addition, the psychobiological predisposition is hypothesized to mediate headache attacks that are precipitated by known events (stress, anxiety, depression, fasting, foodstuffs, menstruation, etc.), as well as headaches that seem to occur spontaneously. Headache attacks in the absence of obvious provocation may constitute the most notable and the most puzzling characteristic of chronic headache sufferers. Although they often experience attacks in association with some specific stressful event rather than in response to it, many of their attacks seem to occur for no apparent reason. This situation can be more frightening and debilitating than the headache attack itself. The position taken here is that the generator (rather than the "cause") for severe headache attacks is found more often in the patient's psychobiological makeup than in the patient's genetics, environment, or biochemistry.

The term *psychobiological predisposition* is far more encompassing in meaning than the more familiar term *genetic predisposition.* The latter term is generally used in reference to an unalterable genetic or constitutional susceptibility. This form of susceptibility is viewed as being independent from psychological factors that contribute to the disorder. However, chronic headache sufferers are not born with chronic headaches. More often than not their condition develops across time, which means that their psychological reactions to the developing symptoms have played a significant role in the development of the disorder. The same can be said of the physiological component of the predisposition. As the disorder increases in severity, more and more physiological systems become involved, and all the systems begin to manifest a kind of autonomy from the environmental events that may have triggered their disorder as occasional headache sufferers. Finally, conceptualizing the predisposition as being largely due to genetic factors has the negative effect of leading patients themselves to believe that there is very little they can do,

...emselves or for their children, to prevent the disorder ...ping. Some patients go as far as to take psychological ... genetic argument, using it as a defense against those who ...wise suggest that the disorder is "all in their head."

...l experts have also strongly reinforced the notion that headache susceptibility is largely due to genetic factors and, by implication, to factors beyond the patient's personal control. For example, Graham (1979) compared the patient's plight to that of a firecracker where "the body of the firecracker is the patient, loaded with genetically explosive powder." Lance (1973) made an even stronger statement on the presumed inverse relationship between genetics and self-control:

> ... laboratory work ... now suggests that migraine is an hereditary recurrent metabolic disturbance. If this be the case, a patient cannot be held responsible for having migraine attacks any more than a woman for having menstrual periods. (p. xii)

It is important that some resolution of the genetic issue be attempted before proceeding further. For example, if Lance is correct in his assertion, then the psychobiological processes outlined in this book indeed will have a secondary significance for understanding the etiology of chronic headache disorders. However, if the order of emphasis is reversed, with psychobiological processes assuming primary status and genetic factors assuming secondary status, then a new approach to the understanding and treatment of chronic headache patients will emerge.

Empirical support for the notion that some form of chronic headache disorders are inherited comes largely from family incidence studies. This literature has focused almost exclusively on migraine headache, with next to no interest in the possibility that muscle-contraction headache may also run in families. If muscle-contraction headache is observed in one or more family members, this is taken as a sign that the family unit is neurotic. If migraine is observed in one or more family members, this is taken as a sign that the disorder is genetically determined. A good example of the double standard that has been used to evaluate family incidence data is provided in the following quotation taken from Sacks (1981):

> An instructive example of "pseudo-hereditary" in the determination of complex psychophysiological reactions is Friedman's finding that not only 65 percent of migraine patients, but 40 percent of patients with

The Psychobiological Model

tension headaches, give a family history of their respective symptoms. It has never been suggested (nor is it likely to be suggested) that tension headaches have a genetic basis, but clearly they are adopted in households where this is the family "style." (p. 151)

The innuendo that parents of children with muscle-contraction headache have somehow transmitted the disorder as a result of their own neurotic headache activity is without empirical support. It also remains to be demonstrated that a child can develop problem headache solely through modelling a parent in pain.

The research that is most often used to support the genetic argument is definitely not as strong as the belief itself. The majority of family incidence studies have been very poorly designed, making it near impossible to make comparisons across the studies (Ziegler, 1977). A rule-of-thumb for appraising the literature is that familial incidence rates seem to vary inversely with the exactness of the methodology used to establish the rates. In one of the earliest studies, Allan (1928) found a history of migraine headache in one or both parents in 349 of 382 migraine patients, yielding an astonishingly high concordance rate of 91.4 percent. Allan did not specify the criteria he employed to diagnose migraine in either the patients or the parents. Moreover, the information on the parents was obtained second-hand from the patients; therefore, the results of this study should be viewed for their historical value only. In another classic study, Goodell, Lewontin, and Wolff (1954) examined the incidence of migraine in the relatives of 119 migraine patients. Although the majority of the data were provided by the patients, a few of the relatives were contacted directly. Approximately 84 percent of the patients had at least one relative with migraine. Of the children having one parent with migraine, 44.2 percent had migraine; of the children having both parents afflicted, 69.2 percent had migraine. Other studies have reported familial incidence rates of headache ranging from 14 percent to 90 percent, but virtually all of these studies suffered from serious design deficiencies (Ziegler, 1977).

Waters (1971) conducted what is probably the best familial incidence study that has been performed to date. Interestingly, he also reported the lowest familial incidence rates of all the studies that have dealt with this issue. In his study, a standardized headache questionnaire was administered directly to 524 immediate relatives of a small random sample of subjects. Some of these subjects had previously been identified as having no headache history of their own, others as having nonmigrainous headaches, and others as having a migraine headache history. The prevalence of migraine was 5 percent and 6 percent in the families of the no-headache and non-migraine headache probands and 10 percent in the families of the probands with migraine. The discrepancy in concordance rates observed in this study from the concordance rates reported in earlier studies is near unbelievable. Clearly, Waters' findings represent a direct challenge to those investigators who insist that migraine has a demonstrable hereditary component.

A more suitable method for assessing the hereditary basis of headache involves the study of concordance rates in identical twins. A few studies are available and, like the findings of the family studies, these results are confusing. The early studies reported concordance values for migraine that ranged from 33 percent to 100 percent for monozygotic twins, and from 0 percent to 40 percent for dizygotic twins (Lucas, 1977). Once again, the majority of these studies were poorly designed, as the criteria for assessing headache and zygosity were seldom specified. Using more rigorous methodologies, recent studies have reported much lower concordance rates from those reported in the early studies. For example, Ziegler, Hassanein, Harris, and Stewart (1975) obtained headache concordance data from a number of twin pairs, all of whom had their zygosity determined by blood grouping in combination with other information (height, weight, physical appearance). They classified the twins on the basis of headache severity rather than on the basis of presence or absence of migraine symptoms. The concordance rate for severe disabling headache in monozygotic twins was observed to be 29 percent (2 of 7 twin pairs), and the concordance rate for dizygotic twins was observed to be 17 percent (2 of 12 pairs). Lucas (1977) reported similar results, with concordance rates of 26 percent and 13 percent for a large sample of monozygotic and dizygotic twin pairs. It is interesting that, although Lucas employed strict criteria to define migraine, his results were quite comparable to those of Ziegler et al., who based their diagnosis on severity criteria. In any case, both these well-designed studies found the genetic component of headache to be quite minimal.

The low concordance rates reported in the more recent family and twin studies are encouraging because they suggest that variables unrelated to genetics are at the basis of headache susceptibility. However, these data are based on averages and may not be too convincing to the headache sufferer who sees headache occurring in one or more immediate family members. In fact, it is the individual case that is often used to dramatically illustrate the hereditary basis of headache. A recent issue of the *National Migraine Newsletter* pro-

The Psychobiological Model

vided a story based on two identical twins who were separa
birth, raised in different environments, and did not see each
until they were thirty-nine years of age. According to the story,
men had married and then divorced a woman named Linda; their
second wives were both named Betty; each owned a dog named Toy;
both had law-enforcement training; both said their favorite school
subject was math; and both vacationed in Florida. Both twins also
suffered from similar headache disorders, which were defined as a
mixture of muscle-contraction and migraine symptoms. A prominent
researcher of twins commented in the article that "when headache is
present in both twin members it suggests that it is not due to environmental but to genetic factors." Does one conclude that divorce,
pet preference, and vacation sites are also determined by genetic
signals?

Articles that illustrate the familial incidence of headache are apparently motivated by an honest desire to "legitimize" some forms of
headache disorders, i.e., to demonstrate that headache is not necessarily due to some form of hidden neuroticism. Unfortunately, there is
a real danger that the consumers of such information may misinterpret
its implications. A headache sufferer with a child who also experiences headaches might conclude that he or she is responsible for the
child's condition and that the child is doomed to a life of pain, misery,
and medication. Such an outcome is not inevitable, even though this
view is often reinforced by popular articles and books. For example,
Oliver Sacks (1981) advised the migraine sufferer to see the disorder
"as part of his biology, his *self*, and, in one way or another, find it
possible to live with it—if not on friendly terms, at least on reasonable
terms." This advice is far too defeatist in nature—children and adults
have the means not to have to live with this disorder on any terms. At
worst only headache susceptibility is transmitted genetically, and
children and adults have a large say in determining the course and
influence of this susceptibility in their lives.

The psychobiological model does not attribute much direct or
current significance to genetic influences. Of course, genetic factors
contribute to the initial occurrence of headache, but once the disorder begins to develop there are far more important variables that
determine chronicity. As will be shown in subsequent chapters, the
most important of these variables are behavioral and not genetic in
nature and concern the headache sufferer's ability or inability to
cope with each successive attack. Like the attack itself, headache
susceptibility is a progressive condition involving a number of complex psychobiological processes.

2
Stress Versus Distress

Few would question that psychological stress is involved in chronic headache attacks. However, there is some controversy with respect to the precise role that stress plays in chronic headache disorders. The majority of research has examined stress and headache within a cause-effect relationship, but there are considerable data suggesting that many headache attacks occur in the absence of psychological stressors. This chapter examines what is known about the relationship between stress and headache, with the objective of presenting a different emphasis on the nature of stress that contributes to the development and maintenance of the chronic headache syndrome. Stress is viewed as a component of the headache disorder rather than as a cause of the headache disorder. Thus, it is proposed that a better understanding of headache susceptibility can be achieved by shifting attention from psychological antecedents to psychological components of the chronic headache syndrome, or, in other words, shifting attention from psychological stress to psychological distress.

The view that psychological stress is an important antecedent of headache attacks was established in the 1930s by Harold Wolff. Wolff was heavily influenced by several psychosomatic theorists who emphasized the role that emotional conflicts and personality characteristics played in mediating between stressful events and the appearance of physical symptoms. Wolff believed that any situation that might elicit rage and resentment, while at the same time preventing the expression of these feelings, was capable of provoking a migraine attack. He saw the precipitating event itself as often being quite trivial, since under other circumstances it would have no effect on these individuals. If conditions were "right," however, the situation would become the "straw that broke the camel's back" and a headache attack would follow. The following case history represents the type of situation that Wolff believed was capable of provoking a headache attack:

> A 30-year-old Italian housewife presented herself at the New York Hospital with a history of almost daily unilateral headache of varying intensity and duration for about two months. Prior to this series of attacks she had had typical migraine headaches every few weeks since adolescence. The present series of headaches paralleled the development of a progressively severe feeding problem in her 4½-year-old daughter. The patient stated that her headaches followed meals with monotonous regularity. The child refused to eat despite the patient's every effort to induce her to do so. At this persistent refusal, the mother would become angry and berate the child violently. Often she would attempt to force food between the child's clenched teeth. Failing this, the mother became so enraged several times, that she assaulted her daughter so violently that the child was left stunned and bruised. Within an hour after such an encounter the patient would develop a high-intensity headache, usually unilateral, which required opiates or ergotamine relief. (Marcusson & Wolff, 1949, p.251)

Most chronic headache sufferers cannot pinpoint situational or psychological stressors that reliably generate their headache attacks. Even if they identify the stressors, they usually view the stressors as exacerbating rather than as causing the headache disorder. For example, Dalsgaard-Nielsen (1965) observed that 68 percent of a group of chronic headache patients recognized that psychological stress could act as a precipitating factor for headache attacks while 32 percent denied this possibility. All of the patients believed that many of their attacks also occurred spontaneously or in the absence of stress. Similarily, Henryk-Gutt and Rees (1973) reported that many headache sufferers, although capable of pointing to events that exacerbated their condition, felt that attacks often occurred in the absence of situational or psychological stress. The researchers also noted that the work and home environments of headache sufferers were not more stressful than the environments of headache-free controls. Andrasik, Blanchard, Arena, Teders, Teevan, and Rodichok (1981) also found that headache sufferers and headache-free controls reported similar exposure to stressful life events as measured by the Social Readjustment Rating Scale (Holmes & Rahe, 1967). Taken together, these studies suggest that stressful situations should be viewed as

ring in association with (and not as causing) headache attacks in
hronic patient.

An illustration of the difficulty of viewing stress and headache onset in a cause-effect fashion was provided by Bakal, Demjen, and Kaganov (1981). In this study, a large number of chronic headache patients were asked to monitor their headache activity on a daily basis, and from these data it was possible to examine the time of day during which their headache attacks typically began. If situational/psychological stress were the principal cause of attacks, one might expect a large number of attacks to have their onset later in the day, after exposure to one or more unpleasant or stressful demands. Such was not the case. As shown in Figure 2.1, the majority of attacks experienced by the patients had their onset upon awakening or within a few hours upon awakening. This was true of patients who had been diagnosed by neurologists as experiencing migraine, muscle-contraction, or combined migraine–muscle-contraction headache symptoms. Given the prevalence of this pattern, it is not surprising that many headache sufferers believe that their attacks occur for no reason whatsoever. Children with problem headache will often state that the attacks begin just when they are about to have a good time, such as playing with a friend, attending a concert, participating in a sporting event, or going on a vacation. In the same vein, adult patients will often ask: "How could my headache be due to stress when I awaken in the morning with a headache already present?" Another question asked by adult patients is: "How could my problem be due to stress, when I am basically satisfied with my job and my life in general?"

Given the patterns of headache onset illustrated in Figure 2.1, it is not difficult to comprehend why chronic headache patients resent being repeatedly told that their disorder is due to stress. Although stress can exacerbate their condition, there is no simple cause-effect relationship between the occurrence of stress and headache onset. It is significant that headache sufferers often complain that the majority of stress they experience is more often the *result* rather than the cause of their headache attacks. The distinction that they are making is between stress and distress. Stress refers to events in the external environment that tax the resources of the person, while distress refers to unpleasant emotional states that arise in response to changes in the external or internal environment. For chronic headache sufferers, living in continual fear that any activity, pleasant or unpleasant, may be interrupted by a headache attack is what is distressing, and usually more so than any concern they may have about the activity itself.

Stress Versus Distress

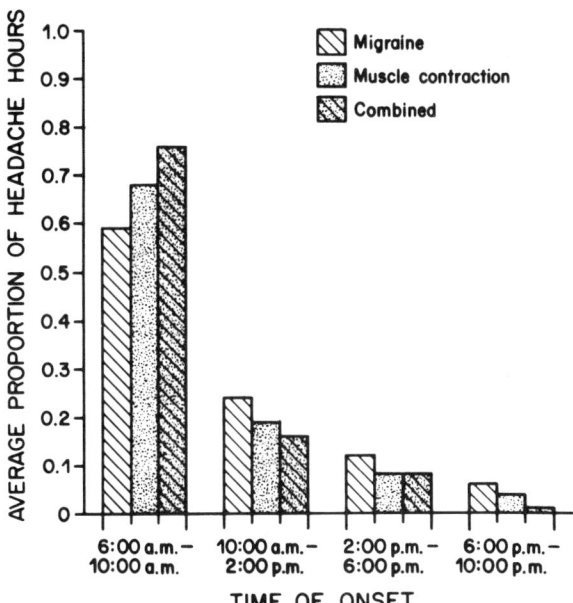

Figure 2.1 Average proportion of headache hours associated with different times of onset (Bakal, Demjen, & Kaganov, 1981). Copyright © 1981 by the American Association for the Study of Headache. Reprinted by permission of the publisher.

The recognition that stress is often a consequence rather than an antecedent of headache attacks is significant because it requires that theoreticians and clinicians rethink their understanding of how stress contributes to chronic headache disorders. Rather than being a static environmental or psychological event, stress becomes an active and dynamic process that influences and is influenced by the very development of the chronic headache syndrome. This view of stress is paralleled very closely by recent developments in stress research. The new look in stress research emphasizes the transactional nature of the phenomenon, and the founder of the approach, R. S. Lazarus, described its implications as follows:

> Psychological stress is now viewed as a general rubric for somewhat different though related processes of person-environment transaction, in which demands tax or exceed the resources of the person. Such stress is neither simply an environmental stimulus, a characteristic of the person, nor a response, but a balance between demands and the power to deal with them without unreasonable or destructive costs.

> Our model of stress is explicitly cognitive-phenomenological, emphasizing how the person appraises what is being experienced and uses this information in coping to shape the course of events. This appraisal of the significance of an ongoing relationship with the environment for one's well-being leads to coping processes consistent with personal agendas. The effects of coping are in turn appraised and reacted to as part of the continuous flow of psychological, social, and physiological processes and events. Stressful commerce with the environment thus involves extensive psychological mediation and reciprocal feedback loops, which cannot be reduced to stimulus and response terms. The nature of stress phenomena therefore requires that any comprehensive model of it be developed within a transactional, process-oriented perspective. (Coyne & Lazarus, 1980, p. 145)

There are several ideas expressed in the above passage that have a direct bearing on the psychobiological model of headache. The main concept that has immediate relevance is the *process-oriented approach,* which Lazarus has advocated as necessary for the study of human functioning. In dealing with stress, he emphasized the necessity of studying the processes that mediate between the person and his or her environment. With the psychobiological model of headache, the emphasis is also process-oriented in nature but concerns the relationship between the patient and his or her symptoms rather than between the patient and his or her environment. In effect, the critical processes that mediate the chronic headache syndrome are found in the relationships between the symptoms experienced, the physiological mechanisms that mediate these symptoms, and the cognitive evaluation of the condition, as the disorder develops across time. The relationships between the cognitive and physiological components of the headache syndrome are seen as bidirectional in nature, with the cognitions influencing the symptoms and the symptoms influencing the cognitions. Thus, a heavy emphasis is placed on the cognitive phenomenological condition of the chronic headache patient.

The emphasis placed on cognitions associated with the headache disorder does not rule out the possibility that situational/environmental factors also play a role in the development and maintenance of chronic headache disorders. Excessively demanding work, social situations, and family situations are expected to characterize chronic headache sufferers as much as similar situations characterize all people who live and function in today's complicated world. Again though, the concern is with trying to formulate an understanding of the phenomenology of the headache sufferer and not with society in general. Most chronic headache sufferers have tested innumerable personal hypotheses concerning the causes of their affliction; surely, if a situational cause of the disorder existed, many would eventually have discovered the connection. The situational-stress hypothesis is more tenable in the developing stages of the disorder since, in the early stages, headache attacks occur more likely in the context of a limited number of events. As the disorder increases in frequency and regularity, however, it is likely that situational explanations begin to make less and less sense to the headache sufferer. For example, many chronic patients who work in stressful careers expect that their headaches will disappear upon vacationing, but this expectancy is usually shattered when the headaches do not cease. The result is usually a ruined vacation accompanied by increased despair and confusion.

What patients and professionals often fail to recognize is that the conditions that lead to a disorder are not necessarily the same conditions that maintain a disorder. Headache may begin as a response to psychosocial stress, but with repeated attacks the psychobiological processes that control the disorder may begin to function relatively independently from such forms of stress. The chronic patient's thoughts are not dominated by problems at work or at home as much as they are by the disorder itself. In fact, the disorder generates (rather than reflects) stress at work and at home, since the patient's employer, friends, and family find it increasingly difficult to understand what is going on. A personal friend of mine suffered from what is called *weekend migraine*, which created a number of personal problems for him. His work was quite demanding, but while at work he was relatively free of headache. However, with the onset of a weekend or a family vacation, he would regularly experience a severe headache attack. His wife became increasingly suspicious and began to accuse him of not loving her and the children any more. The poor fellow eventually decided that the pollen count in his neighborhood was too high, sold his home, bought another, and continued to experience headache attacks as regularly as before. The anecdote also serves to illustrate how a chronic headache sufferer's efforts to understand the disorder can be associated with major disruptions in his or her lifestyle.

The chronic patient's thinking is often heavily oriented towards the disorder itself, a condition that is reflected in the frequent use of statements such as: "Why me, why do I always have headaches?" "Am I being punished?" "I feel guilty about having another headache," "Here we go again," and "This is going to be a bad one."

Chronic headache sufferers have been known to say that, with the onset of any particular headache attack, they experience not only the pain and misery of the present attack but the pain and misery associated with their memories of all previous attacks. The following poem, written by a migraine headache sufferer, appeared in a recent edition of the *National Migraine Newsletter:*

> *I awaken in the morn, with a sickening fear;*
> *The light is too bright, my eye sheds a tear.*
> *I drag my body from my comfortable bed,*
> *But, I can't escape the "aura" surrounding my head.*
> *My husband, so sweet, he knows the drill.*
> *He heads for the cabinet to get my pill!*
> *I lie back down in a state of complete remorse,*
> *What have I done to deserve this painful course?*
> *I yell, "OH NO, NOT TODAY!"*
> *But, I can't control the pain—it's on the way.*
> *My stomach is upset, my eyes a blur,*
> *I've taken too many pills, and begun to slur!*
> *I finally have reached the point that I seek,*
> *My head has just burst—with throbbing at its peak!*
> *I made it, the pain is over,*
> *I'm really not insane!*
> *You must understand—I only suffer from migraine.*

The fact that headache sufferers have negative thoughts and feelings surrounding their disorder comes as no surprise. However, the hypothesis that such thoughts, or what Meichenbaum (1978) has termed *catastrophizing cognitions,* are part-and-parcel of the headache syndrome may indeed elicit some surprise, especially in the patients themselves. Headache sufferers have entertained every other explanatory hypothesis imaginable but never this one.

Headache pain is in many ways a unique type of pain disorder simply because it is not associated with tissue damage. The neurophysiological systems that contribute to the pain are not damaged but are reacting inappropriately. Thus, it becomes more reasonable to assume that the functioning of these systems is inextricably related to the functioning of the cognitive system and that changes in one system will be reflected by changes in the other system. Emphasizing the importance of a cognitive component of the chronic headache syndrome does not mean that headache attacks occur simply because patients "expect" to have attacks, nor does it mean that headache disorders can be reversed magically by the adoption of some naive mind-over-matter philosophy. Headaches are not controlled by cognitions per se, but rather by powerful psychobiological processes that are firmly entrenched in the patient's makeup. However, cognitions represent a powerful tool for both accessing and changing these processes so that headache is no longer a problem.

In the present context, *cognition* is used to refer to both verbal and nonverbal thought processes. In fact, it is more than likely that many of the critical cognitions that mediate headache are nonverbal in nature. Words are actually crude and inadequate labels for many of the neural processes referred to as *thought* (Mahoney, 1980), and this is particularly so for thought related to internal conditions. The familiar complaint, "Words alone cannot convey the pain that I experience," illustrates this point. Patients do talk to themselves about their headaches but the self-talk usually takes place outside their immediate awareness. As a headache begins to develop, for example, most patients cannot recall saying, "Gee whiz, here we go again," but at the same time they can identify with this statement. Therefore, one must be careful not to assume that cognition only refers to thought that is in immediate awareness or that is verbal in nature.

An instructive example of the problems associated with viewing cognitions only in terms of verbal thought comes from a study that examined what children think about headache, i.e., what headache is, what causes headache. Bibace and Walsh (1977) asked groups of children, between the ages of four and thirteen, to respond to a series of health-related questions, one of which was "What is a headache?" The answers indicated very clearly that only the older children were capable of giving adultlike responses, whereas the answers of the younger children followed a logic that was qualitatively different from that used by older children and adults. Very young children (between four and five years) gave answers based on sensory impressions, i.e., in terms of sights and sounds associated with headache via spatial or temporal contiguity. Examples of responses from this age group were: "Headache is from the wind" and "Headache is lying down." Six-year-old children gave what the authors called contagion-type explanations in that they were preoccupied with the link between sensory phenomena and headache attacks: "A headache is from leaning against something." Children between the ages of seven and ten began to distinguish between internal and external events, but their explanations of headache were very concrete in nature: "Headache is when you're noisy and your mother doesn't want you to be"; "Headache gets better when you rub something on your forehead." Ten-, eleven-, and twelve-year-olds gave responses that began to approximate adult understanding of headache in that they understood that the source and nature of the disorder lie within specific physiological structures and functions. A sample response from this age level was: "A headache is from pressure inside your head." It is not until children reach the age of twelve or thirteen that they are able to describe headache with the psychosomatic language that adults use. Illustrative responses from the older children were: "A headache is from problems and aggravations"; "A headache is when you're all nervous and weary"; "A headache is when you drink too much and worry too much." Although not using the word *stress* per se, the older children were capable of identifying stress-related situations and behaviors.

Words are also inadequate for describing the sensory aspect of the headache syndrome. Patients often seem to struggle in their efforts to describe a pervasive internal state that they experience in the absence of pain, as well as in the absence of the stress associated with daily living. Most frequently, the condition is associated with localized sensations from the neck and shoulder region and is described as "feeling continually tight." Other phrases patients use include "constant feelings of pressure" and "feeling like I am always idling too fast." Quite often, the patients do not even notice this condition until its presence is brought to their attention. Whatmore and Kohli (1974) may have been describing this condition when they proposed that excessive *bracing* is at the basis of headache susceptibility: "Bracing efforts consist of signal output from the premotor and motor cortex whereby a portion or all of the skeletal musculature is held partially contracted or 'on guard.'" They also hypothesized that bracing may develop within vascular and autonomic structures that mediate various headache symptoms. Possibly this condition contributes in subtle ways to clinical impressions that some headache sufferers "look like" headache sufferers, even when headache-free.

Coping Styles and Headache Susceptibility

The discussion so far has dealt with the importance of recognizing that cognitive processes associated with headache attacks represent an integral component of the headache syndrome. The next topic is whether or not headache susceptibility and headache severity are also influenced by higher-order cognitive processes, processes usually discussed in the context of personality or coping dispositions. At first glance, it might seem that a headache sufferer's manner of coping with stress in general would influence the coping style he or she would adopt in dealing with head pain. But what does it mean to say, "coping with stress in general?" Do people who successfully cope, or fail to cope, with one stressful event in their lives exhibit similar behavioral patterns with respect to other stressful events? Not necessarily, since a person in a demanding work or home situation might be extremely effective in coping with the requirements of the situation and yet at the same time be totally debilitated by the stress and pain generated by recurrent headache attacks. There is no a priori reason why general dispositional measures of personality or coping should be characteristic of people who have headache disorders. Such measures are usually too abstract and too far removed from the conditions controlling the disorder to be of much theoretical and clinical use.

In a general discussion of the relationship between stress and illness, Cohen and Lazarus (1980) made an important distinction between *dispositional* and *process* approaches to the study of coping. Their observations are most relevant for understanding chronic headache sufferers:

> Coping *dispositions* refer to tendencies of an individual to utilize a particular mode or pattern of coping in a variety of stressful encounters. Research on coping dispositions has focused mostly on narrow coping dimensions ... although broader cognitive styles ... have also been examined. To measure coping dispositions, the tendency of the person to use one or another coping process is usually assessed independently of the stressful event by a questionnaire or a projective technique. This test behavior is treated as a trait measure and considered as a predictor of the coping behavior, observed in some stress situation, such as coping with surgery.
>
> Alternatively, one can study the coping *processes* individuals actually use in coping with a particular stressful situation. The individual's behavior is observed as it occurs in that stressful situation and the mode of coping inferred from it.
>
> One weakness of the dispositional approach is its assumptions regarding consistency in coping behavior. Little evidence exists that there is much consistency in mode of coping from one situation to another.... Situational factors, including demands of the situation, coping options available within it, social supports, and so on, also have important effects on the coping strategies an individual uses.... To the extent these conditions affect the coping processes, trait measures will have limited predictive power. As it turns out, only weak or nonsignificant relationships have been found between measures of coping dispositions and the actual coping behavior observed.... This raises serious questions as to what such coping tests are actually measuring.

> Not only can questions be raised about the consistency of coping from one situation to another, but it is also likely that within a stressful encounter, such as major illness, several different stages of coping may be observed, each with its own pressures leading to the use of different modes of coping.... This variability in coping processes from one time period to another lends support to the argument that dispositional tests of coping provide inadequate measures of actual coping. (p. 223)

From this passage, it becomes evident that an understanding of the psychological component of the chronic headache syndrome is not likely to be attained through the use of general personality measures.

The early headache literature did assign considerable importance to personality variables, but these variables were always presented in an abstract fashion without direct reference to the headache sufferer's beliefs, thoughts, and feelings about the disorder. Wolff (1937) established the notion that there was a *headache personality*, especially in those individuals who experienced migraine headache symptoms. Wolff described migraineurs as being perfectionistic, ambitious, inflexible, reserved, and orderly:

> In general these [migraine patients] were extremely hard working and were endowed with a great deal of energy, "push" and striving. According to their friends they seemed to be tireless in pursuing their goals. In intellectual and creative work this rewarded itself through endless effort to attain the perfect result or flawless data; in others ... the attitude that "everything must be just so." Thus, one housewife called herself a "Dutch cleanser," and her husband jokingly referred to her as a "fanatic with a dust brush," suggestively remarking, "If you would throw away that mop you would probably feel better." (p. 899)

Wolff believed that headache attacks occurred when the underlying conflicts at the basis of these traits were "tickled" by moments of frustration, self-doubt, and self-criticism.

Following the publication of Wolff's clinical observations, numerous empirical efforts were made to establish the significance of pathological personality traits in headache sufferers. Overall, these studies failed to produce strong empirical relationships. The relationships reported were often low in magnitude and nonspecific in nature (Bakal, 1979; Harrison, 1975). In fact, the yield from several decades of personality research was so poor that critics began recommending that the approach be abandoned altogether. At the moment, personality and emotional aspects of headache are receiving little attention and are viewed, at best, as having secondary significance for understanding headache disorders. This is the case even though emotional factors are still cited as the major trigger of chronic headache attacks. The following commentary on the "psychosomatic" status of migraine illustrates the uncertainty associated with psychological variables:

> Emotional disturbance is the commonest single trigger mechanism, and is the most important cause of frequent and severe attacks. There is, however, nothing specific about the emotional stimulus, nor is there a consistent personality type in migraine subjects. Certainly personality reactions and patterns of behavior recur in migraine subjects: a tendency to anxiety reactions, sensitivity to stress, and difficulty in handling aggressive and hostile drives. In this respect, migraine is similar to many other "psychosomatic diseases" without demonstrable pathology but characterized by disorders of homeostasis. In some patients extrinsic physical and biochemical precipitants are prominent and the "psychosomatic element" is slight. In most migraine patients, however, psychologic factors are important but are secondary rather than precipitating etiologic agents. (Pearce, 1977, p. 125)

Dispositional measures can be used much more successfully in headache research *if* they are used with a different objective in mind. Measures need to be used that tap the patient's beliefs, thoughts, and feelings directly related to his or her headache disorder. These headache-related cognitions may or may not be characteristic of the headache sufferer's belief systems in general. In order to better appreciate the change in emphasis that is being recommended, imagine that the usual causal sequence involving psychological variables and headache symptoms is reversed. The situation changes from identifying psychological variables that cause headache to identifying psychological variables that are caused by headache. By reversing the direction of causality in this fashion, it becomes possible to understand how recurrent headache attacks may lead to the development of distress-related beliefs, thoughts, and feelings, which themselves further contribute to a worsening of the headache condition. Since headache sufferers do have beliefs concerning their disorder, and since they also experience considerable distress during painful episodes, the realm of headache-related cognitive activity seems to constitute a rich field of potential exploration.

By shifting the focus of attention to psychological *components* of chronic headache, the task becomes one of examining the experiential aspects of the syndrome and of determining whether or not these aspects influence the course and nature of the symptoms that occur across patients. Demjen and Bakal (1981) conducted an illustrative study of the approach being recommended. They relied on the construct of illness behavior to assess the phenomenological state of headache patients. Mechanic (1962) proposed the concept of *illness behavior* and defined it as "the way in which given symptoms may be differentially perceived, evaluated and acted (or not acted) upon by different kinds of persons." Illness behavior was measured using Pilowsky's Illness Behavior Questionnaire, or IBQ (Pilowsky & Spence, 1975). The IBQ consists of seven scales designed to tap the following psychological components of any illness: (1) general hypochondriasis, (2) conviction of disease, (3) psychological versus somatic perception of illness, (4) affective inhibition, (5) affective disturbance, (6) denial of life problems, and (7) irritability. The IBQ was administered to ninety-four chronic headache sufferers, many of whom had experienced problem headache since adolescence. A headache severity score was derived for each patient and was based on the average number of hours of daily head pain that was reported across a twenty-one-day self-observation period.

The headache patients were found to exhibit illness behaviors similar in nature to the behaviors exhibited by Pilowsky and Spence's general pain patients. At the same time, however, the chronic headache patients were found to differ from the intractable pain patients used by Pilowsky and Spence in several respects. Headache sufferers scored significantly higher on general hypochondriasis and psychological versus somatic perception of illness. Headache sufferers scored significantly lower on disease conviction and denial. These differences suggested that chronic headache sufferers, compared to intractable pain patients, have a stronger psychological focus for their disorder and a greater willingness to discuss psychological problems.

The authors also noted some interesting differences in the IBQ characteristics of headache sufferers themselves. Headache sufferers who experienced continuous or near-continuous pain were found to resemble the intractable pain patients of Pilowsky and Spence along two dimensions of illness behavior. Both groups viewed their pain in somatic as opposed to psychological terms, and both groups scored high on the scale measuring denial of general life problems. It was mentioned that these characteristics are similar to the psychological characteristics often attributed to patients with *psychogenic headache*. Although the diagnostic category is rarely used, one of its primary features is pain that is diffuse and continuous in nature (Weatherhead, 1980). This category of headache is also believed to occur in the absence of mediating physiological mechanisms. A more integrated view would be to assume that there are psychobiological processes that control continuous headache, and that the condition of continuous pain reflects the outcome of the patient's failure to cope with less severe headache that was episodic in nature at an earlier time.

The dimensions of illness behavior assessed by the IBQ were not found to be differentially related to the diagnostic categories of muscle-contraction and migraine headaches or to head pain locations indicative of these diagnostic categories. However, it was demonstrated that as headache activity increased, both muscle-contraction and migraine headache patients showed a tendency to shift from a psychological to a somatic view of their disorder. The shift was also accompanied by an increase in the reported frequency of headaches associated with throbbing and nausea. The observation that patients with the most severe headache activity have a somatic view of their condition may reflect not only their failure to cope with less severe attacks, but may also reflect the appearance of mechanisms that have become increasingly autonomous from specific psychological triggers.

The authors made a final commentary concerning the numerous studies that have attempted to differentiate headache patients in terms of psychopathology. They cited a study by Kudrow and Sutkus (1979) that examined the degree of psychopathology present in several diagnostic categories of headache sufferers, including migraineurs, muscle-contraction headache sufferers, and cluster headache sufferers. Kudrow and Sutkus reported that psychopathology was largely absent in migraineurs and was quite marked in muscle-contraction headache sufferers. Although interesting, their finding might lead to the false conclusion that psychological variables are not critical for understanding patients with migraine symptoms. Demjen and Bakal demonstrated that there are psychological components of the chronic headache syndrome and that these components contributed to the maintenance of the disorder independent of diagnosis. The IBQ study serves to reinforce the empirical approach that is required to develop a holistic understanding of headache sufferers. The critical dispositions, beliefs, and/or high-order cognitive variables that contribute to headache disorders are not to be found in the ad lib use of traditional personality or mental health tests. A more unified approach is to begin developing psychometric measures to assess the cognitive variables that have a direct bearing on the headache disorder.

If re-examined, the traditional psychological research with headache sufferers is actually quite consistent with and supportive of a cognitive approach. It is now generally accepted that headache sufferers are neither more nor less neurotic than the rest of the populace (Philips, 1976). At the same time, however, some interest remains in the potential involvement of what may be called *symptoms of psychopathology*. For example, pain clinics often routinely administer the Minnesota Multiphasic Personality Inventory (MMPI) as a means of assessing the mental status of their patients. The MMPI is used on the grounds that chronic pain patients in general show elevations on several of the subscales (Sternbach, 1974; Swanson, Swensen, Maruta, & McPhee, 1976). Typically, chronic pain patients exhibit marked elevations of the hysteria and hypochondriasis subscales accompanied by moderate elevation of the depression subscale. This particular MMPI configuration has been assigned the name of *Conversion V*. Several studies have demonstrated the presence of a complete or a partial Conversion V pattern in muscle-contraction and migraine headache sufferers (Martin, 1972; Rogado, Harrison, & Graham, 1973).

Elevated scores exhibited by headache sufferers on the hypochondriasis and hysteria subscales of the MMPI may be more indicative of the cognitive correlates of chronic headache than they are indicative of patient psychopathology. The hypochondriasis subscale of the MMPI contains a number of items that can easily be seen as the logical accompaniment of any chronic pain disorder. There are items that deal with headache, stomach complaints, visual and other sensory disturbances, sleep disturbance, fatigue, and dizziness. Many of the same items also comprise the hysteria subscale. Rather than representing exaggerated or unwarranted absorption with bodily symptoms, responses to the MMPI reflect an accurate description by the patient of the misery and suffering that he or she is experiencing. This constitutes a major reversal of the way in which MMPI scores are traditionally used by clinicians, i.e., to imply that pain patients are neurotic and that the neurosis is the cause of their headache condition.

Within a cognitive component framework, MMPI responses can be used to increase our understanding of the psychobiological processes that control chronic headache disorders. By taking the responses at face value, it becomes possible to better appreciate the magnitude of the patient's suffering and also the role that diverse psychological and bodily symptoms play in the overall headache syndrome. For example, Harper and Steger (1978) found that headache *frequency* covaried in a linear fashion with the number of psychological and bodily symptoms reported on the hypochondriasis and hysteria subscales of the MMPI. Kudrow and Sutkus (1979) also found that headache sufferers with more frequent headaches scored higher on hypochondriasis and hysteria than headache sufferers with less frequent headache attacks. The fact that the number of attacks experienced is closely related to the degree of overall psychobiological disturbance represents an important theoretical and clinical observation. It suggests that the cognitive and physiological components of the headache syndrome are inextricably related to each other.

The same argument is applicable to studies that have attempted to link other psychological constructs to headache. To illustrate, some specialists believe that depression is a major cause of chronic headache disorders (Diamond & Dalessio, 1978). Since depression may have replaced anxiety as the mental health symptom experienced with the greatest frequency by the population at large, it is reasonable to assume that physicians will also see, for this reason alone, an increase in the frequency of complaints of depression in their headache patients. Whether depression is the *cause* of headache disorders is another matter. That physicians often believe this to be the case is evidenced by their frequent use of the term *masked depression* to diagnose presenting complaints of headache. Masked depression is a diagnostic label invoked to explain medical patients whose initial complaint is some physical symptom but who upon further examination also admit to being depressed. However, there is no logical reason why admission of depression by a headache patient automatically means that the headache is due to depression. As with stress, most patients would probably argue, if given the chance, that their depression is the result of their uncontrollable headaches.

Depressed headache patients may not even be "depressed" in a clinical sense. In a study of depression in chronic headache sufferers, Couch, Ziegler, and Hassanein (1975) administered the Zung Self-Rating Depression Scale (Zung, 1965) to 265 headache patients. For each patient, they also derived a headache severity score that reflected a weighted average of frequency and duration of headache attacks, as well as perceived disability associated with headache attacks. A positive correlation emerged between the depression scores and the headache severity scores, which might lead one to think that more depressed patients had more severe headaches. But were these patients depressed? Consider the content of the items to which these patients were asked to respond. Representative statements from the Zung scale are the following: "I feel down-hearted and blue"; "I have crying spells or feel like it"; "I have trouble with constipation"; "I get tired for no reason"; "I feel [hope]less"; "I feel that others would be better off if I were dead." These self-statements seem to reflect cognitive and physiological components of the headache syndrome more than they do the "root" cause of the problem. The fact that the cognitive component was found to covary with the severity of symptoms experienced by the patients represents a very significant observation.

In summary, several lines of psychological research point to the importance of headache-related cognitions for understanding headache susceptibility and headache severity. How a patient thinks and feels about the origins of his or her attacks, as well as the painful episodes themselves, is as (if not more) important for understanding the affliction as the particular symptom configuration that accompanies the attacks. This represents a major departure from traditional models of headache disorders, but it is a departure that will increase our understanding of the etiology and treatment of chronic headache disorders. Also, by shifting attention from the psychological antecedents of headache to the psychobiological processes that control headache, it becomes possible to increase our understanding of how variables of quite different levels of abstraction (psychological, physiological, biochemical) interact to produce the headache syndrome. The dualism inherent in the traditional separation of psychological and physiological variables is avoided. The approach parallels very closely the model of pain disorders developed by Melzack (1973). Rather than view psychological variables as secondary to some basic physiological dysfunction, Melzack argued that pain disorders are, potentially at least, under the equal control of sensory, affective, and cognitive variables. This potentiality is more likely with headache disorders than with other clinical pain disorders because headache does not develop in the context of structural damage nor is headache pain usually continuously present. Chronic headache then can be viewed as a unique pain disorder, a disorder that is heavily influenced by the patient's cognitive actions and reactions in dealing with the symptoms themselves.

3
Physiological Mechanisms

Dualistic thinking concerning the etiology of headache disorders receives much of its impetus from biomedical research. In medicine, physiology and biochemistry are seen as "where the action is" and where the basic causes of headache are ultimately to be found. Sympathy for the holistic approach may be found in conversation, but in practice medical researchers remain committed to identifying the neurophysiological/biochemical substrates of headache disorders. That headache disorders have a physiochemical component is without question; the real issue is whether this component exists or can exist independent from the cognitive and sensory variables that were discussed in the previous chapter. This chapter examines the current knowledge of the physiochemistry of head pain and also assesses the extent to which this knowledge is consistent with the psychobiological or severity model.

Two central issues are dealt with in this chapter. The first issue concerns whether or not there is evidence for a physiological component of the predisposition for headache and whether or not this component mirrors the cognitive and sensory components of the disorder that were outlined in the previous chapter. If the physiological literature is found to reflect concomitant processes that occur at the psychological level, then it will no longer be possible to view these as independent events. It will also suggest that headache patients and their symptoms cannot be understood and treated solely from a physiological position. The second issue is whether or not different physiological mechanisms underlie different headache disorders or, more specifically, whether or not migraine and muscle-contraction headache disorders should be viewed as differing quantitatively or qualitatively at the physiological level of analysis. Given the diversity of symptoms that headache patients manifest, there must be a number of different physiological mechanisms that contribute to the symptom differences. For example, the patient who experiences dull and aching head pain will most likely not have the same physiological substrate for his or her disorder as the patient who experiences throbbing pain preceded by visual disturbances. However, both patients may exhibit commonalities in other physiological systems, and these commonalities may explain why both patients are susceptible to chronic headache. Also, the presence of physiological differences may be better understood as reflecting quantitative rather than qualitative differences in terms of the degree of involvement of physiological systems that contribute to the chronic headache syndrome.

Vascular Mechanisms

The majority of physiological research has been directed towards identifying vascular mechanisms that are associated with headache attacks. Interest in vascular mechanisms is due to the widespread interest in migraine headache pain and, within the traditional medical model, migraine is presumed to be a vascular disorder. A schematic of the vascular changes that are believed to precede and accompany migraine attacks is presented in Figure 3.1. Vascular changes are hypothesized to take place both within the skull (intracranial) and outside the skull (extracranial). The working physiological model of migraine is that the attack is preceded by a state of arteriolar narrowing or vasoconstriction. This state defines the pre-headache or prodromal phase of the attack and is followed by the painful phase that is believed to develop in response to vasodilation of the extracranial arteries and smaller vessels in the temporal region of the head.

The notion that migraine head pain is associated with extracranial vasodilation was first demonstrated in a classic study by Graham and Wolff (1938). They administered ergotamine tartrate, a vasoconstrictive substance, to subjects during the headache phase of a migraine attack and simultaneously recorded extracranial vasomotor activity from the superficial temporal and occipital arteries. Some subjects (the exact number was not specified) showed decreases in pulse amplitudes that were interpreted as due to the vasoconstrictive effect of ergotamine. Some patients also showed a decline in the subjective

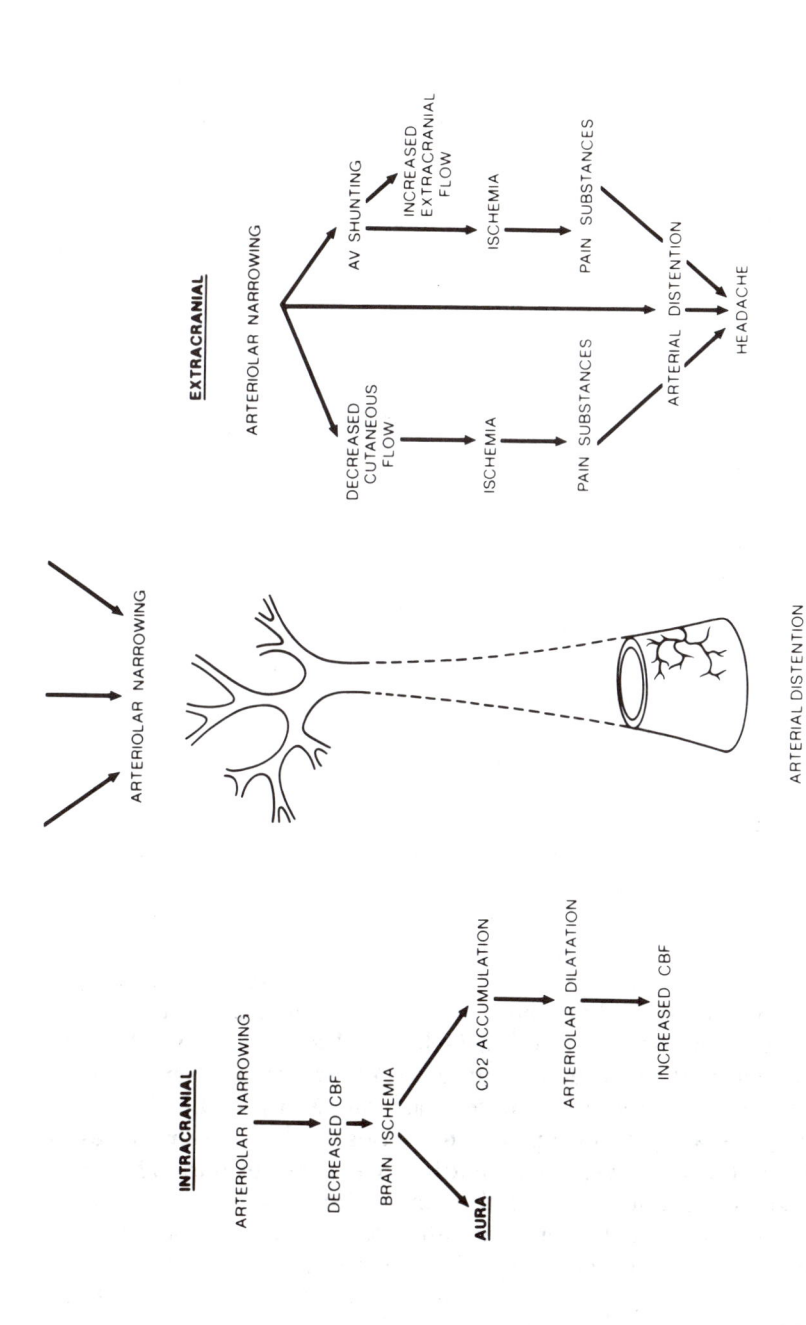

Figure 3.1 Vascular changes in migraine (Edmeads, 1979). Copyright © 1979 by the American Association for the Study of Headache. Reprinted by permission of the publisher and J. Edmeads.

intensity of headache, with the decline mirroring the changes in the pulse wave amplitudes. Unfortunately, Wolff failed to relate statistically the two indices of headache activity, but he claimed that, if the amplitude of the pulsations decreased slowly in response to ergotamine, the headache likewise decreased slowly. If the pulse amplitude dropped precipitously, the headache was ended promptly.

Wolff (Dalessio, 1980a) used similar drug-induced change procedures to test the hypothesis that the painful phase of migraine is preceded by extracranial vasoconstriction and also that accompanying visual symptoms are associated with intracranial or cerebral vasoconstriction. Wolff did not have access to the technology that is currently available for studying cerebral blood flow, so he tackled the problem by administering drugs that were known to influence both the extracranial and intracranial vasculature. For example, he had one patient inhale amyl nitrate, a vasodilator of both cranial and cerebral vessels, during a period when the patient was experiencing a marked preheadache visual disturbance. Immediately following the inhalation, the visual disturbance disappeared, only to return after the amyl nitrate had worn off. In another study, Wolff used carbon dioxide and oxygen to produce vasodilation of the cerebral arteries. Migraine patients were required to inhale mixtures of carbon dioxide and oxygen during the prodromal phase of their attack (when vasoconstriction is presumed to be present) and during the headache phase (when vasodilation is presumed to be present). When the carbon dioxide–oxygen mixture was inhaled during the preheadache phase, it was associated with an "immediate and lasting disappearance of the visual disturbance and the expected headache did not follow." The inhalation of vasodilative air mixture had no predictable effect when the headache was already present (i.e., the pain did not increase or lessen in intensity).

Wolff performed many other experiments to support the vasoconstriction-vasodilation hypothesis of migraine, and a complete summary of his work is presented in Dalessio (1980a). It should be mentioned that Wolff's research, although extensive, was at the same time often presented in a biased fashion. Many of his published observations were based on selected cases, and he never addressed the issue of how general these findings were. For example, he stated that ergotamine injections reliably aborted migraine attacks, but yet it is known today that many migraine patients do not benefit from taking ergotamine-based drugs. The same criticism applies to his observations with amyl nitrate and carbon dioxide: some patients showed the expected responses and others did not.

Wolff was also theoretically committed to viewing migraine and muscle-contraction headaches as separate disorders, with each disorder having a separate etiology. Consequently, he most often collected psychophysiological data from one or the other diagnostic group without exploring the possibility that similar physiological phenomena may occur in both groups. Before examining the more current vascular literature, it is instructive to examine one more study reported by Wolff (Tunis & Wolff, 1954). This study is important because it represents one of the few times that Wolff collected vascular *and* musculoskeletal data from the same patients. The patients were muscle-contraction sufferers rather than migraine headache sufferers, and the data were obtained during a session with the pain present and during a session with the pain absent. During the headache session, the EMG measure showed, in the words of Tunis and Wolff, "a tenfold increase in amplitude of action potentials." Matching the EMG increase was a significant decrease in the amplitude of the recorded pulse waves, which was interpreted as a sign of vasoconstriction. The vasoconstriction may have been present outside of the headache state as well, since several of the patients showed reduced pulse amplitudes in the headache-free condition. This latter observation may be most significant because it implies that some headache sufferers possess a physiological susceptibility for the disorder that is manifest in both the musculoskeletal and vascular systems. Wolff failed to pursue this possibility because of his certainty that muscle contraction and migraine headache were qualitatively different disorders. From a severity perspective, however, these data suggest that the patient who experiences vascular and muscle-contraction symptoms may have evolved into the difficult position of continually being undermined by two physiological systems, the musculoskeletal and the vascular.

The more recent research on the extracranial vascular changes associated with headache has not been very supportive of Wolff's preliminary observations. Wolff made most of his observations by placing transducers over the larger extracranial arteries (e.g., superficial temporal), but there is a growing suspicion that the vascular changes that contribute to headache, if present, must be mediated by changes in smaller vessels of the head. Such changes may not even be discernible from transducers placed over the large extracranial arteries. This suspicion is supported by some unpublished observations from our laboratory. In this research, ultrasonic transducers were used to improve the recording technique of blood flow activity in the superficial temporal arteries. Transducers were affixed bilaterally and pulse velocity waves were obtained from a large sample of chronic headache sufferers, both with the symptom present and with the symptom absent. Although the pulse-wave tracings were extremely reliable and reproducible from one session to the next, there were no characteristics to the wave forms that differentiated the headache-nonheadache sessions nor the headache patients from healthy controls. The hemodynamic changes associated with headache susceptibility and headache attacks are probably quite subtle and varied in nature, at least more so than those implied to occur in Wolff's photograph of a migraine patient with a bulging temporal artery during a headache attack (Dalessio, 1980a, p. 79).

Using the ultrasonic doppler method, other investigators have had more success, but more in terms of identifying persistent vascular anomalies rather than in terms of identifying vascular concomitants of the headache state. Otis, Smith, Kroll, Krasny, Seltzer, and Dalessio (1979) recorded pulse-wave velocity from the supraorbital temporal artery while simultaneously compressing the superficial temporal artery, as shown in Figure 3.2. This manipulation was carried out in a large number of migraine patients during sessions with the symptom present and during sessions with the symptom absent. A normal response to the manipulation is an increase in blood flow to the orbital artery following compression of the superficial temporal artery. A decrease in orbital flow is interpreted as a sign that the internal carotid artery, which normally receives the additional flow to the ophthalmic artery, is in a state of occlusion or vasoconstriction. A small percentage of the migraine patients showed evidence of vasoconstriction, which when present was not necessarily specific to the presence of head pain. Several patients showed signs of an abnormal response over a number of sessions in which they were headache-free.

Using the same application of ultrasonic transducers and arterial compression, Kudrow (1979a) found signs of persistent vasoconstriction in cluster headache patients. Cluster headache is a rare form of pathological headache and was so named because the attacks have a clustering character both within and across days (Kudrow, 1979b). The pain is unilateral in nature and generally specific to the eye and temporal region. Kudrow recorded pulse-wave velocity from probe sites placed over the supraorbital and frontal arteries on both sides before and after temporal artery compression. When symptom-free, 70 percent of the cluster patients showed a reduction in ipsilateral flow to this maneuver when compared to contralateral flow. The decrease in ipsilateral flow was even greater when the patients were tested with pain present. This study again points to the presence of a perva-

Physiological Mechanisms 33

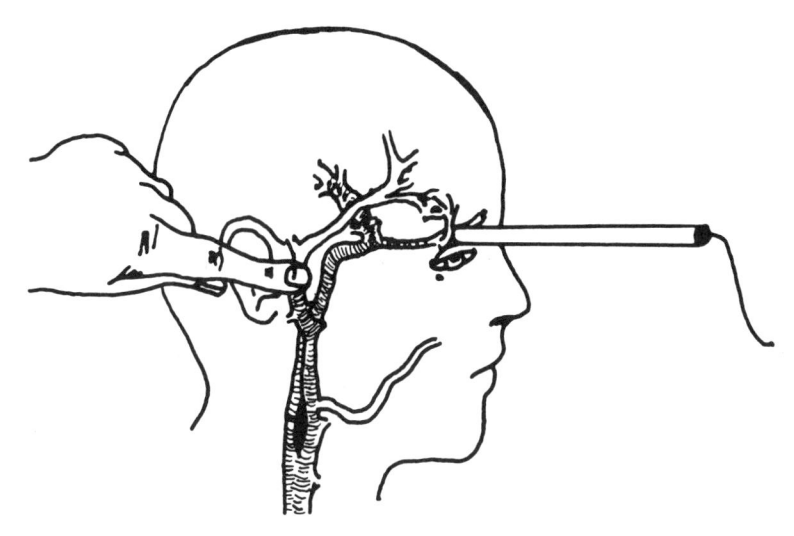

Figure 3.2 Doppler Ophthalmic Test. Supraorbital artery is monitored with a directional Doppler flowmeter, while blood flow through the superficial temporal artery is obliterated by manual compression. Copyright © 1979 by the American Association for the Study of Headache. Reprinted by permission of the publisher and S. M. Otis.

sive vasoconstrictive state that may render the patient susceptible to headache attacks. The observation that the vasoconstriction was specific to one side of the head attests to the high degree of physiological individuality that exists within some headache sufferers.

Musculoskeletal Activity and Headache Susceptibility

Until very recently, it was widely believed that the vascular changes that contributed to headache disorders occurred independently from changes in the musculoskeletal system. As mentioned previously, the independence notion had its beginnings with Wolff, who was so committed to the migraine–muscle-contraction dichotomy that he saw no necessity of making direct physiological comparisons of migraine and muscle-contraction patients. In the past few years, however, several researchers have demonstrated that heightened musculoskeletal activity is present in both diagnostic groups and that this activity can be detected whether or not pain is actually present. Within the severity model, this activity represents a significant component of the headache predisposition and is at the basis of complaints of persistent feelings of tightness and pressure that are found to characterize the chronic headache patient.

The first study to demonstrate the presence of heightened musculoskeletal activity in chronic headache sufferers was conducted by Pózniak-Patewicz (1976). She recorded EMG activity from the neck and temporal regions in patients who had been diagnosed as muscle-contraction headache sufferers, migraine sufferers, and headache-free controls. For some headache patients, the recordings were obtained without the symptom present, and for others with the symptom present. Both headache groups were found to exhibit greater EMG activity in the symptom-free condition than the no-headache controls. Somewhat surprisingly, the migraine patients manifested *greater* EMG activity than did the muscle-contraction patients under both experimental conditions. Pózniak-Patewicz attributed no etiological significance to her finding that both muscle-contraction and migraine headache patients showed evidence of persistent muscle spasms. In fact, she concluded that muscle spasms most likely are a consequence of both types of headaches and have no etiological significance for understanding either one of them.

In a direct physiological comparison study, Bakal and Kaganov (1977) found results quite similar to those observed by Pózniak-Patewicz (1976). Using surface recording electrodes (Pózniak-Patewicz used needle electrodes), they compared the neck and forehead EMG levels of migraine and muscle-contraction patients during a session with severe headache present and during a session with headache absent. EMG levels were also monitored in a group of subjects who claimed never to have experienced headache. The migraine patients manifested significantly higher frontalis EMG levels during the nonheadache condition than either the muscle-contraction patients or the headache-free controls. In addition, both headache groups had significantly higher neck EMG levels than the headache-free controls. Neither headache group showed a significant change in EMG activity from the nonheadache to the headache condition.

A third study found that migraine patients exhibited greater EMG activity in the symptom-free condition than did muscle-contraction patients. Philips (1978) monitored frontal, temporal, neck, and trapezius EMG levels of patients with migraine headache, muscle-contraction headache, and headache of mixed symptomatology, and of no-headache controls. The measures were obtained during a rest period, and only the frontal EMG resulted in significant

Physiological Mechanisms

differences between groups. Migraine patients demonstrated the greatest frontal EMG levels, followed by patients with mixed symptomatology, muscle-contraction headache patients, and finally the no-headache controls. Philips also observed that EMG levels correlated poorly with the intensity of pain experienced during a headache attack, a finding that has been noted by others (Bakal & Kaganov, 1977; Holroyd, in press).

Not all studies have found heightened EMG activity to be characteristic of headache sufferers in general. In a recent study, Anderson and Franks (1981) recorded both frontal and forearm EMG activity from subjects with muscle-contraction headache and migraine headache, and from headache-free controls. The measures were obtained across two separate recording sessions, and there were no signs of consistent differences between the groups. This was true of EMG baseline or resting data, as well as of reactivity data obtained in response to physical and psychological stress. The authors concluded that there is no reliable relationship between headache susceptibility and EMG activity. Their conclusion may be accurate but not necessarily because musculoskeletal activity is not present in headache sufferers. Especially when recorded with surface electrodes, the EMG is at best only a crude index of muscle tightness and tenderness. For example, it is possible to palpate muscle tenderness and yet not detect any concomitant surface EMG abnormalities in some subjects. Strictly speaking, it is also meaningless to compare headache patients in terms of *microvolt levels* obtained from a particular muscle site because the microvolt readout is influenced by variables other than myopotentials from muscles in the immediate vicinity of the electrodes. According to Basmajian (1976), the EMG from forehead surface electrodes "reflects the total or global EMG of all sorts of repeated dynamic muscular activities down to about the first rib—along with some postural activity and nervous tension overactivity."

Of course, it is dangerous to persist with an hypothesis that is supported only by data obtained with a measure that is defined as a poor one. However, there is additional evidence that heightened muscle activity plays a subtle but powerful role in severe headache disorders. Tfelt-Hansen, Lous, and Olesen (1981) conducted a thorough assessment of muscle tenderness in migraine patients using palpation rather than EMG activity. Pericranial tenderness was evaluated by palpation in twenty-six muscles and tendon insertions. When possible, symmetrical muscles were palpated simultaneously. The presence or absence of tenderness was determined on the basis

CASE 3

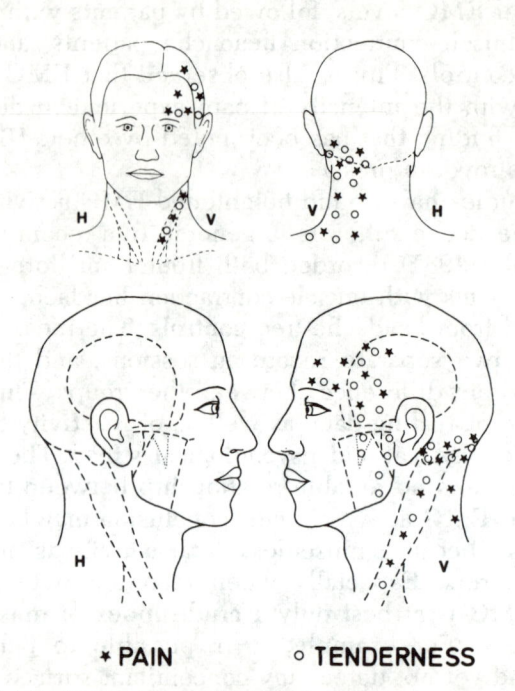

* PAIN   ○ TENDERNESS

Figure 3.3 (a) Patient with unilateral pain location during common migraine attack (stars). The localization of tenderness (open circles) is almost identical to that of pain. (b) Patient with bilateral pain location during common migraine attack. Pain (stars) and tenderness (open circles) coexist in

of the patient's verbal pain complaint, grimacing, or withdrawal. The palpation data were obtained from the patients during an acute attack of migraine. Muscle tenderness was found to be present in all fifty patients. The muscles most often affected were sternocleidomastoid, anterior temporal, neck, and shoulder muscles. Interestingly, the affected muscles mediate tonic rather than dynamic functions, which points to the presence of a pervasive condition. The sites of tenderness and pain corresponded highly, except for the forehead. Although this region was often associated with pain, it was seldom associated with tenderness. The authors hypothesized that forehead pain may be referred from tenderness in the sternocleidomastoid muscle (an observation that has implications for the use of frontal EMG measures). Figure 3.3 contains two examples of the correspondence that occurred between the pain sites and the tenderness sites. The patients were also injected with either saline or lidocaine (a

Physiological Mechanisms 37

CASE 38

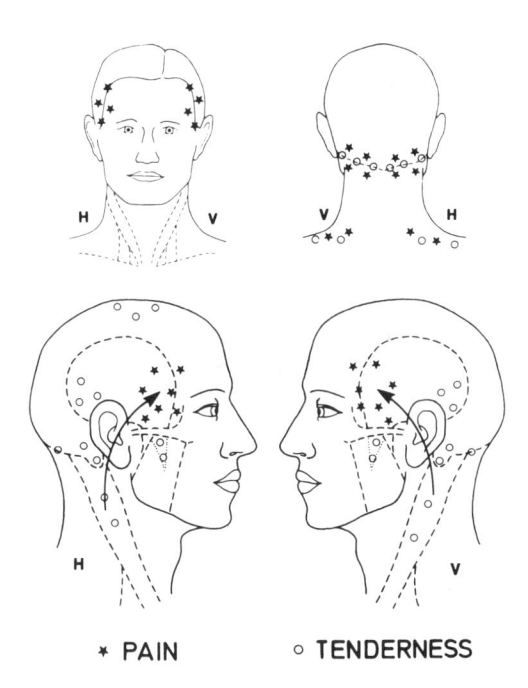

* PAIN   ○ TENDERNESS

most areas. In the posterior temporal muscle and the sternocleidomastoid muscle there is tenderness without pain. Latter muscles may project pain to temples and brow (arrows), which explains forehead pain without tenderness. Copyright © 1981 by the American Association for the Study of Headache. Reprinted by permission of the publisher and J. Olesen.

potent local anesthetic agent) in regions of greatest tenderness. Both substances were associated with equal amelioration of pain, which suggested that muscle and tendon tenderness may be part of an important musculoskeletal mechanism that leads to the onset of migraine headache attack.

The presence of musculoskeletal activity in chronic headache sufferers, in particular those diagnosed as migraineurs, will not come as a surprise to experienced clinicians. In fact, Wolff (Ostfeld & Wolff, 1958) studied EMGs of the scalp and neck muscles in patients with migraine headaches and found evidence for considerable muscle contraction in these patients during the headache episode and during headache-free periods. Rather than interpret this activity as an important component of the migraine syndrome, Wolff decided that it was indicative of another form of headache disorder, unrelated in origin to the mechanisms that generated the migraine attack:

There is another type of head pain which occurs in migraine patients. It may be present concomitantly or in the interval between migraine attacks. Such headache is nonpulsatile, of low or moderate intensity, and may last for days, weeks, or years. The individual feels as if he has a hat on when he has none; that his neck is in a cast; that his shoulders are sore; that if he could be rubbed he would feel more comfortable. Action potentials recorded from the head and neck muscle during such a headache indicate vigorous contraction. (p. 1503)

Several studies have provided data that support the presence of a musculoskeletal component of the headache predisposition. In some studies, the relationship between musculoskeletal activity in the nonheadache condition was linearly related to the severity of symptoms experienced during the headache state. That is, sustained muscle activity apparently becomes more pronounced as one moves from no-headache cases to muscle-contraction cases to migraine cases. It was also noted that this activity may be accompanied by persistent sensations of tightness and pressure. Generally, these sensations have been overlooked by physicians and patients in their search for the causes of chronic headache attacks.

Cerebral Blood Flow Studies

The understanding of what takes place inside the skulls of headache sufferers (physiologically speaking) began with the development of noninvasive techniques for studying intracranial or cerebral blood flow. A radioactive material, such as isotope-labelled Xenon (^{133}Xe), is injected directly into the internal carotid artery, or alternatively, is inhaled through a face mask. The radioactive material has a short half-life and is administered in doses small enough to avoid risk to the patient. Scintillation detectors placed on the outside of the head (Figure 3.4) monitor the rapidity with which the radioactive material is washed through the blood vessels. The more rapid the disappearance of the radioactivity, the greater is the rate of intracranial blood flow. There is also a method for ensuring that the observed changes in flow are not due to changes in the extracranial vessels in the immediate vicinity of the detectors. Xenon generates both X-ray activity and gamma activity, and because X-ray activity has less penetrance, it is believed to reflect extracranial rather than intracranial blood flow. Given this to be the case, it becomes possible to mathematically remove the X-ray effect from the total effect, leaving a pure estimation of intracranial blood flow. The measurement of intracran-

Physiological Mechanisms 39

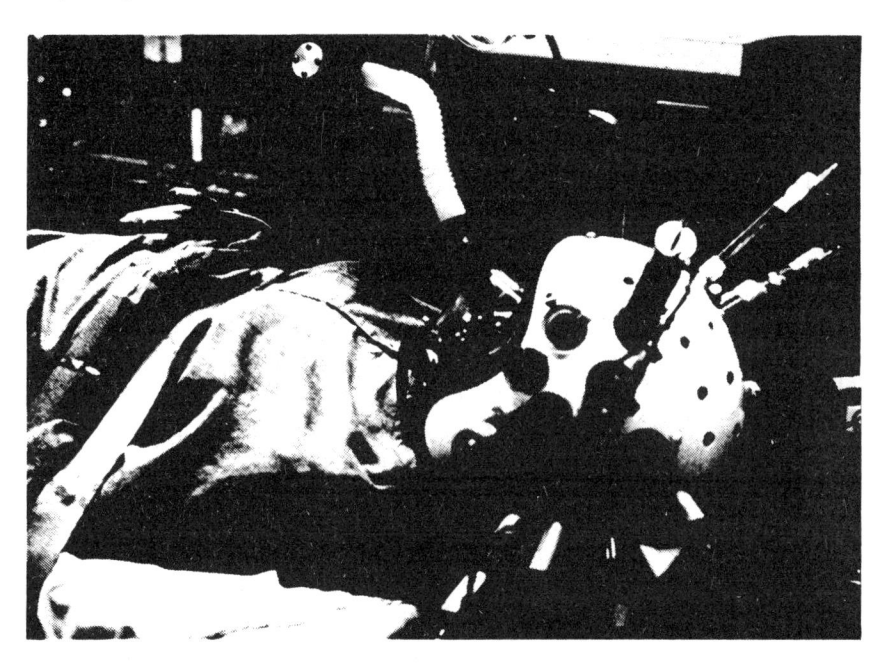

Figure 3.4 Photograph of patient with migraine headaches undergoing ^{133}Xe cerebral blood flow measurement in the laboratory of John Stirling Meyer, M.D., Chief, Cerebrovascular Research, VA Medical Center, Houston, and Professor of Neurology, Baylor College of Medicine. Reprinted by permission of J. S. Meyer.

ial flow at any particular detector site or combination of sites is referred to as an index of *regional cerebral blood flow (rCBF)*.

The technology associated with the measurement of rCBF has the potential for answering a number of important theoretical questions. First, do changes in rCBF mirror the vasoconstriction/vasodilation sequence that is hypothesized to occur in the extracranial vessels? Second, are changes in intracranial blood flow specific or general in nature? That is, during the painful episode, do blood flow changes occur in regions of the brain thought to control the pain and associated symptoms, or do the changes occur throughout the cerebral vasculature? Third, are changes in cerebral blood flow detectable only in the headache state, or, as was observed with the extracranial vasculature, are there reductions/increases in rCBF during headache-free periods as well? Finally, are changes in rCBF specific to migraine headache sufferers, or are similar changes also present in muscle-contraction headache sufferers?

In one of the earliest studies with this technique, O'Brien (1971) recorded rCBF from two scintillation counters placed on either side of the head of eighteen migraine patients. For some of the patients, the rCBF was measured during the prodromal phase, while for others the rCBF was measured during the headache phase. During the prodromal phase, a reduction of 23 percent in rCBF occurred and the reduction was generalized to both hemispheres. There was no evidence of localized rCBF changes that would account for the appearance of localized prodromal symptoms (e.g., visual disturbance in either the left or right eye). O'Brien postulated that the specificity of prodromal symptoms may be a reflection of predetermined structural idiosyncrasies that exert their influence against a background of generalized vasoconstriction. During the headache phase, there were slight increases in rCBF (of the magnitude of 8 percent) that did not match the large decreases observed during the prodromal phase.

Other studies have found marked decreases in rCBF during the prodromal phase of migraine. Simard and Paulson (1973) obtained rCBF data from a group of thirty-two females who reported experiencing unilateral left-sided pain during their headache attacks. An injection procedure was used and rCBF was measured only for the left side of the brain. When the patients were not having headaches, the rCBF was within normal limits, but when the prodrome was present the rCBF decreased by about 50 percent of the normal value. Mathew, Hrastnik, and Meyer (1976) reported a 36 percent reduction in rCBF during the prodrome in three migraineurs and found that the reductions were diffuse and bilateral even though the patients had specific neurological symptoms indicative of localized ischemia of the occipital and parietal lobes.

Localized occurrences of cerebral vasoconstriction during the prodrome have been detected, but these seem to represent the exception rather than the rule. Skinhøj and Paulson (1969) reported rCBF data on one patient who experienced tactile and motor disturbances in the right hand accompanied by speech and language difficulties, which taken together are symptoms believed to be mediated by the parietal and temporal lobes. Cerebral blood flow was reduced throughout the brain during the prodrome, but the greatest reduction was apparent in the parietal and temporal lobes.

There is some evidence that cerebral blood flow increases during the headache phase of a migraine attack. A normal rCBF is taken to be approximately 50ml/100gm/min. Mathew, Hrastnik, and Meyer (1976) found the rCBF of migraineurs to be within normal limits with the symptom absent; with headache present, however, the rCBF increased to 56.8ml/100gm/min. Sakai and Meyer (1978) also found the rCBF of migraineurs to be normal when the patients were headache-free but to increase substantially with the onset of pain. Interestingly, in some patients the increase in blood flow persisted up to two days beyond the termination of the headache attack. Cluster headache patients also showed marked increases in rCBF during headache attacks. Unlike migraineurs, however, they quickly returned to preheadache rCBF values following the termination of their attacks.

Three of the four questions raised at the opening of this section have been answered. With the onset of the headache attack, there is evidence that cerebral vasoconstriction occurs during the prodromal phase and changes to cerebral vasodilation during the headache phase. The vasoconstriction/vasodilation sequence is apparently general in nature, involving the entire cerebral cortex. There is no evidence that migraine headache sufferers show signs of persistent cerebral vasoconstriction outside the migraine attack, corresponding to the evidence suggesting the presence of persistent cranial vasoconstriction. It is possible that between headaches the cerebral flow is normal while the cranial flow is constricted. However, it must be mentioned that Sakai and Meyer provided data that were inconsistent with the observations made earlier concerning cranial vasoconstriction. Using data based on the X-ray component of Xenon administration, they found that the extracranial blood flow of migraineurs was within normal limits.

Do muscle-contraction headache sufferers show any signs of cerebral blood flow changes that parallel the observations made with migraine headache sufferers? Both Mathew et al. and Sakai and Meyer included muscle-contraction patients in their rCBF studies. No evidence was found for the existence of cerebral blood flow increases or decreases during the pain of muscle-contraction headache. At the same time, no effort was made to assess the severity of pain experienced by the muscle-contraction patients during the recording sessions. It is possible that these subjects were experiencing a mild and nonspecific headache attack. This alone would account for the physiological differences that were demonstrated to exist between muscle-contraction and migraine headache sufferers. If the muscle-contraction patients had been experiencing a severe attack, they too may have experienced changes in cerebral blood flow, both in anticipation of pain and in the presence of pain.

Another strong possibility is that the rCBF changes observed during severe headache attacks are more a reflection of the psychological component of the pain than the physiological mechanisms leading to the pain. For example, Sakai and Meyer observed that a few of their muscle-contraction headache patients showed increases in rCBF during the headache attack and that the increases were more likely to occur in the patients who were showing signs of anxiety and tension. It may be that increases in rCBF represent a generalized defensive response to any noxious or painful event. Ingvar (1976) described an experiment in which significant increases in rCBF followed the application of a painful stimulus to the thumb. He saw the relevance of this observation for understanding the migraine attack to be as follows:

> When the subject with migraine starts to experience headache, this pain increases the cerebral metabolism, which in turn augments the cerebral vasodilatation—and the pain—still further. Thus a positive feedback circuit is set up as a vicious circle in which the vasodilatation causes pain, which in turn increases the vasodilatation and the headache grows steadily worse. (p. 5)

This statement reinforces the idea that cerebral blood flow changes during the headache state are not reflective of some basic physiological dysfunction per se. The nature and magnitude of the rCBF response may in large part be determined by the magnitude of the psychological distress associated with the pain of headache. Distress may be what exacerbates the feedback loop and what ultimately causes the affliction to snowball beyond the patient's control. Whether similar psychological processes mediate the vasoconstriction that occurs during the prodrome (e.g., anticipation of pain, worry, dread) is unknown but the possibility is worth exploring. The rCBF studies may not have led to the localization of primary pain mechanisms, as some had hoped, but they have demonstrated quite convincingly just how massive and encompassing the physiological changes associated with headache can be.

Instability of the Autonomic Nervous System

Severe headache attacks are associated with symptoms mediated by the autonomic nervous system, the most frequently experienced autonomic symptoms being nausea and vomiting. The presence of such symptoms has led some theorists to speculate that migraine headache is a disorder of the autonomic nervous system (Bruyn, 1980). At one time migraine was viewed as an autonomic disorder with headache constituting only one of the symptoms associated with the disorder. Migraine has also been called a form of *autonomic epilepsy* (Lennox, 1960), the implication being that it constituted a functional neurologic disorder more similar in nature to epilepsy than to muscle-contraction headache. The autonomic instability hypothesis may have originated with clinicians who observed that adult headache sufferers often reported childhood histories of gastrointestinal instability associated with symptoms such as cyclical vomiting, nausea, travel sickness, and fainting (Selby & Lance, 1960; Smith, 1937).

Laboratory analogues of autonomic instability have met with limited success in demonstrating this phenomenon in chronic headache sufferers. Physiological researchers have attempted to empirically demonstrate autonomic instability by studying reflex vasomotor responses to heat stimuli. The application of heat to the body trunk is normally followed by reflex vasodilation in the extremities. Appenzeller, Davison, and Marshall (1963) compared the reflex vasomotor responses in the hands of migraine subjects with similar responses in the hands of headache-free subjects. The body trunk was heated with light bulbs, and blood flow through the hand was measured with a venous occlusion plethysmographic technique. All of the control subjects showed signs of vasodilation, but eight of ten migraine patients failed to show the effect. Other investigators have been unable to replicate this finding. Hockaday, MacMillan, and Whitty (1967) and French, Lassers, and Desai (1967) found no difference in peripheral reflex vasomotor change in migraineurs compared to nonheadache control subjects in response to thermal stimuli. In a careful review of studies that used the heat-induced reflex procedure, Morley (1977) concluded that most investigators failed to use proper experimental design procedures, making it impossible to adequately assess their findings. For example, only one study controlled for the long-term effects of ergotamine usage, a drug which is known to abolish the vasodilation reflex, and this study found no evidence of vasomotor reflex dysfunction in migrainous individuals.

Psychologists have examined vasomotor reflex responses in headache sufferers, using auditory rather than heat stimuli to induce the reflex. Bakal and Kaganov (1977) administered a series of white noise stimuli to migraine and muscle-contraction headache sufferers, with the objective of studying the patients' cranial vasomotor (superficial temporal artery) responses with an orienting/defensive response framework. According to the Russian literature (Sokolov, 1963), the orienting response is associated with cranial vasodilation, while the defensive response is associated with cranial vasoconstriction. North American researchers have typically reported the cranial orienting response to consist of initial vasoconstriction followed by vasodilation (Cohen & Johnson, 1971).

Bakal and Kaganov found little evidence that headache sufferers differed from each other (muscle-contraction vs. migraine) or from headache-free controls. There was a slight tendency for the pulse velocity responses in the superficial temporal arteries to decrease in the headache groups and to increase in the controls, but the difference was marginal.

Price and Clarke (1979) used a learning paradigm to study vasomotor abnormalities in migraine headache sufferers. Rather than record from the temporal arteries, they recorded vasomotor activity from the finger, on the assumption that this peripheral measure would reflect, if present, a generalized vasomotor abnormality. The learning paradigm consisted of a differential classical conditioning procedure that involved the presentation of conditioned stimuli (CS) consisting of a series of 500 db tones of either 400 Hz or 1200 Hz. One tone was designated the positive conditioned stimulus (CS+) for half the subjects, and the other tone designated the CS+ for the remaining subjects. For the conditioning phase of the study, the CS+ was followed by an unconditioned stimulus of white noise (90 db). The negative conditioned stimuli (CS−) were not paired with the white noise. The data indicated that headache-free controls exhibited the expected differential response to the two stimulus conditions, showing digital vasoconstriction to the CS+ stimuli and vasodilation to the CS− stimuli. On the other hand, the migraineurs exhibited vasoconstriction to both classes of stimuli, which the authors interpreted as evidence of migraineurs' failure to develop an appropriate conditioned response.

Except for the Price and Clarke study, there is little empirical evidence for the notion that chronic headache sufferers possess either a generalized vasomotor dysfunction or an unstable autonomic nervous system. However, the fact remains that many headache sufferers do experience an assortment of symptoms that are mediated by the autonomic nervous system (nausea, vomiting, diarrhea, dizziness, fainting spells). Researchers may have to realize that laboratory contrivances that deal with reflex responses to laboratory stimuli (heat, light, noise) have little to do with the complex processes that control symptoms involving the autonomic nervous system. With this awareness, it should become possible to devise better laboratory analogues, analogues that mirror the full range of psychobiological processes that contribute to the development of such symptoms.

The Origin of Pain

The psychobiological model of headache does not view pain as a discrete event, separate from the other components of the headache syndrome. A patient's thoughts and feelings are as important for understanding the pain experienced during a headache attack as are the localized physiochemical events that allow the patient to specify where it is that he or she hurts. The position taken is consistent with the cognitive behavioral view of pain, which holds that pain is a multifaceted experience involving cognitive, behavioral, and physiological events (Genest & Turk, 1979). It is encouraging that current physiological research with pain mechanisms is supportive of the holistic model of pain (Liebeskind & Paul, 1977). A number of discoveries, including the endorphin systems, have made it clear that experienced pain can no longer be studied as reflecting the simple transmission of a pain impulse from the injured region to a pain center in the brain. It is now known that the transmission of such impulses is modulated extensively by excitatory and inhibitory mechanisms located in the periphery, spinal cord, brainstem, and cerebral cortex, and the suspicion is that this modulation takes place before the experience of pain occurs. Although specialized mechanisms for pain do exist, no mechanisms in isolation are sufficient to account for the pain experience.

In his *gate-control theory*, Melzack (1973) must be credited with foreseeing the present theoretical and empirical developments in pain research. He prophetically recognized that pain was not the same as other sensations mainly because pain, unlike other sensations, had a strong affective or emotional quality. Melzack defined pain as:

> a perceptual experience whose quality and intensity are influenced by the unique past history of the individual, by the meaning he gives to the pain-producing situation and by his "state of mind" at the moment. We believe that all these factors play a role in determining the actual pattern of nerve impulses that ascend from the body to the brain and travel within the brain itself. In this way, pain becomes a function of the whole individual, including his present thoughts and fears, as well as his hopes for the future. (p. 48)

Beecher (1959) is also to be credited for recognizing that there is not necessarily a one-to-one relationship between peripheral injury and pain experienced. After observing a large number of wounded soldiers in World War II, he reached the conclusion that pain is not necessarily determined by tissue damage alone. In his famous quotation, he indicated that how one appraises an injury can determine the degree and quality of pain experienced:

> The common belief that wounds are inevitably associated with pain, and that the more extensive the wound the worse the pain, was not

supported by observations made as carefully as possible in the combat zone ... The data state in numerical terms what is known to all thoughtful clinical observers: there is no simple relationship between the wound per se and the pain experienced. The pain is in large part determined by other factors, and of great significance here is the significance of the wound. (p. 165)

The pain experienced during headache attacks is determined by other factors in addition to biochemical events occurring at the site that hurts. With this observation in mind, the discussion now turns to a brief examination of the biochemical component of the chronic headache syndrome. The vast majority of theorizing and research in this area has been directed towards the biochemistry of migraine. Because research on migraine seldom includes muscle-contraction sufferers as a control group, there is little evidence to indicate that the biochemical alterations associated with migraine attacks also do not occur during muscle-contraction attacks. At least some of the biochemical findings associated with migraine have been observed in muscle-contraction headache sufferers (Rolf, Wiele, & Brune, 1981).

Migraine attacks are presumed to be mediated by changes in the extracranial and intracranial circulation. However, it is recognized that vascular changes alone are not sufficient to produce pain because similar vascular changes produced through exercise or exposure to heat are not experienced as painful. There is at least one additional link in the chain of events that leads to pain, and this link is believed to be biochemical in nature. Dalessio (1974) hypothesized that the vasodilation associated with headache, unlike the vasodilation associated with exercise and heat, is accompanied by the appearance of a localized inflammatory reaction in the walls of dilated vessels. The reaction is believed to be mediated by one or more vasoneuroactive substances, such as histamine, tyramine, neurokinin, 5-hydroxytryptamine, and prostaglandins (Bruyn, 1980). Although some or all of these substances may play a role in head pain, it is safe to say that none has as yet acquired the status of being a "headache enzyme."

One of the strongest advocates of the biochemical approach to the study of headache is Sicuteri (1976). Sicuteri developed a biochemical theory of headache that postulates that head pain is due to central biochemical dysnociception, a condition resulting from a failure in the patient's brainstem to adequately turn over 5-hydroxytryptamine or serotonin. According to Sicuteri, serotonin normally acts as a pain-inhibiting mediator within the central nervous system, and headache sufferers are unable to produce sufficient quantities of this mediator. Serotonin (a potent vasoconstrictor of scalp arteries) has received more theoretical attention in headache research than the other vasoneuroactive substances, and prior to Sicuteri's hypothesis it was believed to exert its effects primarily in the periphery. It was presumed that serotonin levels dropped prior to the onset of head pain and that the drop was associated with extracranial vasodilation, which then led to the experience of pain. In a study of plasma serotonin levels of migrainous subjects during migraine attacks as well as headache-free periods, Curran, Hinterberger, and Lance (1965) found that in 80 percent of the subjects serotonin levels were lower during headache. The fall was found to occur at the onset of the migraine attack and to persist for most of the duration of the headache. There are other studies that have demonstrated decreases in serotonin levels during headache attacks (Sjaastad, 1975). However, not all patients have shown the expected fall in serotonin levels. Furthermore, the observed changes in serotonin levels could have been a consequence rather than a cause of the headaches.

As an overview, it appears that there are multiple physiological and biochemical systems involving the entire nervous system that contribute to headache susceptibility and headache attacks. In spite of the complexity of the problem, there is a rudimentary knowledge of some of the systems involved, and this knowledge provides support for several working hypotheses. For example, heightened musculoskeletal activity contributes to headache susceptibility in patients who experience a variety of symptoms during headache attacks. With more severe headache disorders, there is a good possibility that increased sympathetic tone and cranial vasoconstriction are present during headache-free periods. There is also some evidence that severe headache disorders are associated with cranial vasoconstriction during the preheadache phase and cranial vasodilation during the headache phase. There is no strong evidence that patients diagnosed as muscle-contraction headache sufferers exhibit physiological characteristics that are qualitatively different from those exhibited by migraine headache sufferers. On the contrary, it appears that the physiological differences among headache sufferers are quantitative rather than qualitative in nature, with the physiological systems becoming more involved and encompassing as the disorder increases in severity.

4
One or More Kinds of Headache?

In medicine, headache symptoms are considered to operate independently from the headache sufferer's psychological reactions to the symptoms. Symptoms are used to determine the particular pathophysiological disturbance involved (e.g., whether the disorder is musculoskeletal or vascular in origin). The patient's reactions to the symptoms, especially in the case of migraine symptoms, are not seen as directly influencing the nature of the pathophysiology. The psychobiological approach views symptoms differently. The patient's symptoms are seen as being inextricably related to the patient's psychological reactions to these symptoms. Regardless of the patient's specific symptomatology, chronic headache is seen as a progressive disorder with a symptomatology that becomes more extensive across repeated attacks. Migraine then is seen as a severe form of headache that often develops, rather than as a disease that the patient is born with or acquires. The same view is held for severe forms of muscle-contraction headache.

A significant component of the present thesis is that significant symptom similarities exist across headache sufferers, especially headache sufferers who are often differentially diagnosed as suffering from migraine or muscle-contraction headache. These similarities are not simply academic since they point to critical psychobiological processes that are involved in the etiology and maintenance of chronic headache attacks. This chapter examines the existing headache symptom literature in order to determine whether symptom differences among headache sufferers can be better understood along a continuum of severity rather than in terms of the traditional diagnostic system. In some respects, the traditional distinction between muscle-contraction headache and migraine headache has acquired the status of dogma. In science, a model is revised or abandoned when it fails to account adequately for all the data. On the other hand, a dogma requires that discrepant data be forced to fit the model or be excluded (Engel, 1977).

Not only medical specialists believe in the validity of the muscle-contraction–migraine dichotomy, but a large number of headache sufferers also share this belief. This is especially true of patients who seem to find a perverse solace in being diagnosed as migraine headache sufferers. It is as if the diagnostic label frees them from the suspicion that their headache might have a psychosomatic origin. In the eyes of many headache sufferers, migraine is a legitimate headache disorder, whereas muscle-contraction headache is not. For this reason, patients will often defiantly assert that they suffer from migraine and *not* from headache. A patient in our clinic liked to emphatically state, "I came by my headache *honestly*—my father had migraine and my grandfather had migraine." Some family practitioners have been known to use the diagnostic label of "migraine" solely to avoid hurting their patients' feelings and to avoid having them think that they suffer from some psychiatric disorder.

Headache sufferers deserve sympathy and admiration for having to contend with academic and layman "experts" who view their problem as being inconsequential and one that would disappear if they could simply "get their act together." Until recently, headache was not considered to be a serious medical disorder by medicine, unless of course the headache proved to be symptomatic of some underlying organic problem. Harold Wolff and his associates deserve recognition for changing this attitude. Because of their pioneering efforts, a large number of medical scientists are now committed to advancing the understanding of headache causes and control. However, there is the problem that some scientists and patients feel that a disorder must have a biochemical cause in order to be legitimate. It is partly for this reason that medical specialists adhere to the distinction between migraine and muscle-contraction headache since migraine, unlike muscle-contraction headache, is assumed to have a biochemical origin.

As will be demonstrated, there is a strong empirical argument for altering the current approach to headache diagnosis. Not only do the traditional migraine symptoms fail to cluster in accordance with accepted definitions of migraine, but muscle-contraction symptoms also appear to be an integral component of what is commonly referred to as the migraine syndrome. More often than not, muscle-contraction and migraine symptoms occur concomitantly and, although symptom differences do exist among headache sufferers, the differences are not adequately captured by the muscle-contraction–migraine dichotomy. It seems far more appropriate and accurate to view these symptoms along a continuum of severity, with increasingly severe attacks being accompanied by more frequent and encompassing symptoms (musculoskeletal, vascular, autonomic). Before developing this argument further, it is instructive to examine the traditional system of headache classification and the data that are used to support this system.

Classification of Headache

In 1960 the National Institute of Neurological Diseases and Blindness established a committee with the mandate to formalize headache diagnosis. The committee's solution was to devise, on the basis of clinical consensus, a system of classification that contained fifteen categories of headache (Ad Hoc Committee on the Classification of Headache, 1962). For purposes of discussion, Diamond and Dalessio (1978) reduced the fifteen categories to three general groupings of headache disorders: (1) traction and inflammatory headache, (2) vascular headache, and (3) muscle-contraction headache (Table 4.1). The first grouping, traction and inflammatory headache, is beyond the scope of this book. This grouping refers to headaches that are indicative of some organic disease of the skull and its components, including the brain, meninges, blood vessels, eyes, ears, teeth, nose, and sinuses. The diagnosis and treatment of headache would be much simpler were it possible to differentiate organic headache from nonorganic headache on the basis of symptom configuration alone. Unfortunately, this is not the case. (The reader is referred to Diamond and Dalessio for a discussion of the organic factors in headache.)

Under the grouping of vascular migraine headache, Diamond and Dalessio included classic migraine, common migraine, and two variants of complicated migraine called hemiplegic and ophthalmoplegic migraine. The latter two variants are quite rare and refer to the presence of neurologic symptoms (slight paralysis of one side of the body, paralysis of the ocular muscles) that accompany and persist

Table 4.1 Classification of Headache

Vascular Headache	Muscle Contraction Headache	Traction and Inflammatory Headache

Migraine
  Classic
  Common
  Hemiplegic
  Ophthalmoplegic
	Depressive equivalents and conversion reactions	Mass lesions (tumors, edema, hematomas, cerebral hemorrhage)

Cluster (histamine)	Cervical osteoarthritis	Diseases of the eye, ear, nose, throat, teeth
Toxic vascular Hypertensive	Chronic myositis	Infection Arteritis, phlebitis (Cranial neuralgias) Occulsive vascular disease Atypical facial pain TMJ disease

From Diamond & Dalessio, 1978. Copyright © 1978, The Williams & Wilkins Co., Baltimore. Reprinted by permission of publisher and S. Diamond.

beyond the headache period. Toxic vascular headache refers to all conditions that produce vascular headache as part of their symptom complex, the best example being fever. Cluster headache is a rare variant of vascular headache, with its incidence being less than 1 percent in the general headache population. It was so named because the attacks have a clustering character, both within and across days (Kudrow, 1979b). The afflicted individual may be entirely headache-free for a number of months and then suddenly begin to experience very severe attacks of pain. The pain is unilateral, nonthrobbing, and located in the eye region. It may be accompanied by tearing, pupillary constriction, and nasal stuffiness of the affected side of the head. The attacks occur with a frequency of one to three times a day, each lasting for approximately forty-five minutes. They may occur in this fashion for several weeks or months only to suddenly cease and be followed by a long remission period. In some instances, there is no remission period.

The grouping of muscle-contraction headache replaced the more familiar label of tension headache, possibly because of the negative and misleading connotations associated with the latter diagnostic label. Diamond and Dalessio listed the major variant of muscle-contraction headache as headache due to depression and conversion reactions. This represents their particular theoretical emphasis more than it does the decision of the Ad Hoc Committee. Also included under the muscle-contraction category were headaches due to degenerative joint diseases and diseases of muscle tissue. Muscle-contraction headache is rarely due to disease per se, and it is also difficult to determine if the presence of a degenerative disease is the actual cause of muscle-contraction pain or whether the disease simply accompanies the muscle-contraction pain. Once organic causes of muscle-contraction headache are ruled out, the next step is to separate this form of headache from migraine headache.

How did the Ad Hoc Committee propose to differentiate muscle-contraction headache sufferers from migraine headache sufferers? The first diagnostic criterion the committee used was based on differences in the nature and location of pain that occurred during muscle-contraction and migraine headache attacks. The pain of muscle-contraction headache was defined as dull and aching in nature and bilateral and occipital/frontal in location. The architects of the system recognized that the distinction was more of a relative rather than of an absolute kind, as it was obvious to them that patients seldom experienced pure muscle-contraction or migraine head pain. Possibly for this reason, they placed greater emphasis on the presence/absence of associated symptoms, both prior to the onset of head pain and during the actual period of head pain. The Ad Hoc Committee's distinction between classical and common migraine was made to formalize the position that only a classical migraine attack is preceded by an aura or prodromal phase. However, most diagnosticians do not make the distinction between classical and common migraine, but they do consider prodromal symptoms as being paramount for the diagnosis of migraine. The most dramatic prodromal symptoms involve the visual system, with the patient being frightened by the sudden appearance of blind spots (scotomata), zigzag patterns (teichopsia or fortification spectra) as shown in Figure 4.1, or flashing colored lights (photopsia). Such symptoms usually disappear with the onset of head pain, but the patient may now report the appearance of new symptoms such as nausea, vomiting, light sensitivity, and hypersensitivity to noise.

Nausea and vomiting are probably the main symptoms that diagnosticians use to separate migraine from muscle-contraction headache. In fact, Olesen (1978) has recently proposed that a revision be made to the Ad Hoc Committee's definition of migraine, with greater emphasis being placed on the presence of nausea and/or vomiting:

> Common migraine is a disorder characterized by recurrent attacks of headache of unknown etiology. The headache must be associated with

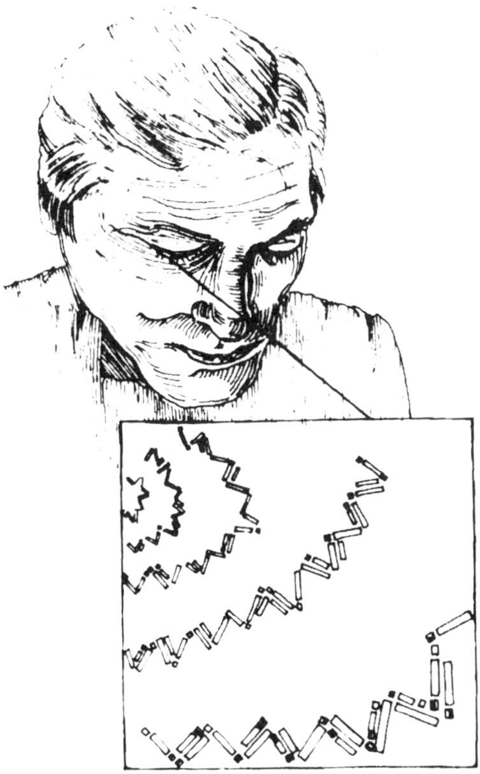

Figure 4.1 An illustration of teichopsia or fortification spectra—zigzag pattern resembling a fort (Diamond & Dalessio, 1978). Copyright © 1978, The Williams & Wilkins Co., Baltimore. Reprinted by permission of the publisher and S. Diamond.

> gastrointestinal dysfunction (anorexia, nausea or vomiting) . . . or with at least two of the following symptoms: unilateral pain location, pulsating quality of pain, phonophobia, photophobia, or other visual disturbances. (p. 270)

Muscle-contraction headache is not accompanied by autonomic symptoms or by any other associated symptoms. In fact, one of the major criticisms of the traditional classification system is that muscle-contraction headache is defined mainly by exclusion of symptoms that are taken as indicative of migraine headache (Philips, 1977).

An additional criterion for separating muscle-contraction and migraine headaches has emerged since the Ad Hoc Committee laid down its definitions of these two headache disorders. The criterion is based on the frequency with which the attacks occur and therefore does not refer to any etiological mechanism per se. Headache attacks that possess migraine characteristics (auras, nausea, vomiting, unilaterality) are cited as occurring less frequently than attacks that resemble muscle-contraction headache. As a rule of thumb, migraine is seen as occurring at a rate of once or twice per month, while muscle-contraction headache is seen as occurring, at least in the chronic patient, on a daily or near-daily basis. Some researchers have taken to operationalizing this criterion in their patient selection procedures. For example, Kudrow and Sutkus (1979) defined migraineurs as patients who experienced "recurrent attacks occurring no more often than once a week." Muscle-contraction patients were defined as patients who experienced "constant or almost constant pain."

A final criterion that is used to differentiate muscle-contraction headache from migraine headache relates to their presumed different patterns of onset. Muscle-contraction headache is presumed to develop slowly, usually in response to stress, whereas migraine headache is presumed to begin suddenly and without provocation. Lance (1973) views the paroxysmal nature of migraine as the critical defining feature of the syndrome:

> In view of the wide variation in clinical symptoms, it is remarkable that there is usually little difficulty in the diagnosis of migraine, the reason being the repetitive paroxysmal nature of the disorder. Difficulty arises when the frequency of attacks is such that migraine recurs almost daily or where migraine is superimposed upon daily tension headache. In both instances it may be difficult to sort out the vascular component from the background of nervous tension or depression. (p. 94)

As indicated previously, it is this paroxysmal feature of migraine that makes some theorists believe migraine is closer to epilepsy in origin than it is to muscle-contraction headache. The paroxysmal nature of some headache attacks is discussed further in a later chapter that deals with concerns associated with the psychobiological model of headache.

All headache sufferers do not experience the same symptoms. On the contrary, each headache sufferer represents a unique individual in terms of the particular configuration of symptoms that he or she experiences. Chronic headache sufferers exhibit marked variation from each other, not only in terms of the frequency and duration of their headache attacks but also in terms of the location and quality of pain they experience. For some patients, the pain is highly localized, involving the region of the eye or the top of the head. For others, the pain is more generalized, involving a number of regions of the neck and head. Some patients show marked variation within themselves, experiencing what appear to be qualitatively different symptoms on different occasions. Even within a single attack, the location, intensity, and quality of pain may change dramatically, beginning as a bilateral, dull, nonspecific ache and developing into a unilateral, throbbing pain.

Given this variability in headache symptoms, headache classification must constitute a diagnostic nightmare for most physicians. Only recently have some physicians begun to verbalize their concerns in trying to separate patients into the categories of muscle-contraction and migraine headaches. Ziegler (1979) used the following case study to illustrate the heterogeneity of symptoms experienced by headache sufferers:

> A 35-year-old woman had episodic severe headaches beginning at age eight, usually associated with nausea and vomiting, and often with vertigo and faintness. In her twenties, she began to have bouts of moderate headache, two or three times weekly, present on awakening in the morning, persisting throughout the day, and only partially relieved by analgesics. The bouts were usually separated by three to six months of headache-free periods. In the year prior to examination at the clinic, the patient had had a headache almost every other day, present on arising in the morning. These headaches tended to be retroorbital, on the right side, not associated with nausea and vomiting, relieved by rest and a mild analgesic-sedative combination. The woman had a worrisome disposition, worked "under pressure," but tended to have the bouts of headache as often when she was on vacation as during working periods. She had had three attacks with visual scotomata followed by hemicrania, nausea, and vomiting. Physical, neurologic, and laboratory examinations were negative. (p. 445)

The variability in symptom patterns exhibited by this patient throughout her history of headache is not atypical.

Empirical Observations of Headache Symptoms

Surprisingly few studies are available that have attempted to empirically assess the validity of the Ad Hoc Committee's diagnostic system. Moreover, based on the available studies, it is apparent that the classification of headache patients into muscle-contraction and migraine headache sufferers is not as simple as the classification of headache itself. Several studies have demonstrated that chronic headache patients cannot easily be described as suffering from the traditional symptom clusters of either muscle-contraction or migraine headache. These same studies suggest that headache symptoms can be better understood along a continuum of severity and, in this sense, are consistent with the physiological observations made in the previous chapter.

In 1954 Friedman, von Storch, and Merritt presented in tabular form their clinical perceptions of the symptoms experienced by 2000 patients who had been diagnosed as suffering from migraine and muscle-contraction headaches. This study is often cited as confirming the majority of the diagnostic features of muscle-contraction and migraine headaches as outlined by the Ad Hoc Committee. A summary of their clinical impressions is presented in Table 4.2. In actuality, few of the symptoms provided a clear differentiation between muscle-contraction and migraine headaches. The best headache discriminations occurred with the symptoms of throbbing pain, unilateral pain, and nausea/vomiting. At least 50 percent of the patients from the migraine group were observed to manifest these symptoms, while, at most, 10 percent of the muscle-contraction patients were perceived to experience these symptoms.

Throbbing pain, unilateral pain, and nausea/vomiting are traditional migraine symptoms, and at first glance the Friedman et al. data present a case for symptom differences between muscle-contraction and migraine headache sufferers. However, there is a strong possibility that the investigators' preconceptions influenced their ratings of the symptoms. In fact, the very presence or absence of these three migraine symptoms determined whether the investigators in their initial diagnosis of the patients viewed the presenting headache as muscle-contraction or migrainous in nature. In addition, no effort was made to summarize the degree of symptom overlap that occurred in the two diagnostic groups, although the authors acknowledged that many of the patients suffered from both muscle-contraction and migraine headache attacks. However, the attacks were viewed as independent events.

The picture is far less consistent when empirical rather than clinical methods of classification are employed. Using a multivariate approach to classification, Ziegler, Hassanein, and Hassanein (1972) demonstrated little concordance between the symptoms reported by patients and the symptoms that define migraine. They administered

Table 4.2 Comparison of the Symptoms of Patients Diagnosed as Having Migraine and Muscle-Contraction Headaches

	Percentage of Patients with Diagnosis	
	Migraine	Muscle-Contraction
Positive family history	65	40
First headache occurred when less than 20 years old	55	30
Prodrome present	60	10
Frequency		
constant or daily	0	20
less than once per week	60	15
Duration		
constant or daily	0	20
from one to three days	35	10
Throbbing	80	30
Unilateral	80	10
Associated with vomiting	50	10

From Friedman, A.P., von Storch, T.T.C., & Merritt, H.H. Copyright © 1954, by *Neurology*. Reprinted by permission of the publisher.

a symptom checklist of twenty-seven items to 289 headache sufferers. A factor analysis of the twenty-seven symptoms yielded seven factors, none of which singly contained the variables thought of as diagnostic of the migraine syndrome. In fact, the classical symptoms of migraine were represented by three factors. Visual and motor preheadache symptoms characterized the first factor, while symptoms of nausea before and during the headache state represented the second factor. Unilateral pain, pain above the eye, and scalp tenderness characterized the third factor. The relative independence of the factors indicated that the three clusters of symptoms were not statistically correlated with each other, as might be expected if migraine headache formed a discrete diagnostic category. Although this study is important, factor analytic solutions to classification must be regarded with caution. Factor analytic solutions are generally unreliable and arbitrary, depending as they do on the particular technique used and the patient/symptom population sampled. A practical disadvantage of factor analytic solutions is that the resultant symptom clusters, in addition to being near impossible to remember, generally do not point to solutions for understanding the individual patient and his or her symptoms.

Physicians who are satisfied with the traditional classification system might take comfort in the fact that no system of headache classification is likely to yield *perfectly* homogeneous categories of headache disorders. However, the system should at least be capable of identifying a diagnostic group who experiences symptoms that are *largely* independent from the symptoms experienced by other groups. For example, Diamond and Dalessio (1978) stated that about 70 percent of migraine headaches are associated with unilateral pain. And yet, unilateral head pain does not occur in conjunction with other migraine symptoms more frequently than bilateral head pain. Philips (1977) examined the degree to which unilateral and bilateral head pain were differentially related to the migraine symptoms of nausea/vomiting and preheadache visual disturbance. According to the traditional diagnostic system, unilateral head pain should occur more frequently than bilateral head pain in the presence of these migraine symptoms. Using data from 597 headache patients, Philips reported that nausea/vomiting and preheadache visual disturbance occurred more frequently in conjunction with bilateral pain than with unilateral pain.

Hunter and Philips (1981) used a second approach to examine symptom similarities and differences between muscle-contraction and migraine headache sufferers. Headache patients who had been differentially diagnosed as experiencing muscle-contraction or migraine headache were asked to describe the quality of pain that was typical of their attacks. The patients were asked to respond to the McGill Pain Questionnaire (Melzack, 1975). The MPQ consists of twenty scales of pain quality descriptors that are categorized into three categories: sensory, affective, and evaluative. Muscle-contraction and migraine patients were virtually identical in their responses to the sensory scales. However, some of the affective scales differentiated the two groups. Migraine patients made more frequent use of affective descriptors such as sickening, nauseating, blinding, and sharp to describe their headache attacks. Approximately 80 percent of both diagnostic groups rated tension as being associated with their disorder. These data indicate that headache patients do differ in the quality of pain experienced. However, it is still reasonable to assume that the different symptoms experienced by patients cluster around a particular point on a severity continuum.

Blanchard, Andrasik, Arena, and Teders (in press) used a psychophysical scaling procedure to examine the quality of pain experienced by different diagnostic groups of headache sufferers. Following a measurement procedure developed by Tursky (1976), they had headache sufferers scale a number of adjectives that are frequently used to describe pain. Fifteen adjectives were chosen to reflect the intensity component of pain: extremely weak, just noticeable, very weak, weak, mild, moderate, uncomfortable, strong, intense, very strong, severe, extremely strong, very intense, intolerable, and excruciating. Eleven adjectives were used to reflect the reactive component of pain: bearable, tolerable, uncomfortable, distracting, unpleasant, distressing, miserable, awful, unbearable, intolerable, and agonizing. Patients used two psychophysical scaling techniques to indicate the magnitude of each pain descriptor. Along with a headache-free control group, four categories of headache patients were used in the study: muscle-contraction, migraine, combined, and cluster. The groups did not differ in the ratings of the intensity descriptors, but they did differ in the ratings of the reactive descriptors. All three headache groups rated the reactivity descriptors higher than the headache-free controls. In addition, the headache sufferers who experienced more severe headaches rated the reactivity descriptors higher than patients whose headache attacks were thought to be less severe. Cluster headache patients rated the reactivity adjectives highest, followed by patients with either migraine or combined headache, and muscle-contraction headache. The study demonstrated that patients with severe headache attacks mean something different when they describe their condition as "intolerable" than patients with less severe headache. Further research with this innovative technique may yield information concerning the manner in which the reactivity dimension of pain is related to other properties of the headache syndrome.

Advocates of the traditional diagnostic system do not demand that every feature of migraine need be present in order to establish the diagnosis. The critical features that must be present vary from diagnostician to diagnostician as well as from researcher to researcher. There are no agreed-upon rules as to how many and what kind of migraine symptoms must be present in order to make a headache sufferer a migraine headache sufferer. Some medical specialists demand that throbbing pain be present in all cases and that the pain be accompanied by at least two of the following characteristics: unilateral pain, associated nausea, visual or sensory aura, cyclic vomiting in childhood, and family history of migraine. Others demand that some other symptom, such as nausea or gastrointestinal disturbance, always be present in combination with one or more of the traditional migraine symptoms. This situation is unsatisfactory because it allows the same diagnostic label to be applied to patients who may differ greatly in the symptoms associated with their disorder. In agreement with this position, Olesen (1978) stated that the current approach to defining migraine is too vague and too variable to form a satisfactory basis for research. "Is it migraine if a patient has attacks of bilateral pressing pain with nausea, but no visual disturbances? Is it migraine if a patient has daily aching diffuse headaches and, on top of that, episodes where the pain intensifies, becomes throbbing in quality, and associated with nausea and vomiting?"

Symptoms vary considerably among patients, both within and across headache attacks. To compensate for this variability, researchers often ask patients to describe only their *worst* or most *typical* headache. This form of assessment can be quite misleading since it does not give due recognition to the full range of symptoms that headache sufferers are known to experience. As a first step in evaluating the full range of headache symptoms experienced by chronic headache sufferers, both across and within headache attacks, Bakal and Kaganov (1976) devised a self-observation record that permits the daily monitoring of headache activity and thus avoids the problems associated with having patients recall their symptoms. The *headache frequency record* is prepared in the form of a postcard and permits the patient to systematically observe and describe his or her headache activity as it develops. A sample of a completed record is presented in Figure 4.2. The data obtained from the card also provide a means of determining the extent to which muscle-contraction and migraine headache symptoms occur as discrete events. Patients who experience more than one kind of headache often state that "my last attack was not one of my worst," or "I have had several headaches recently, but I have not had a migraine for weeks." There is no question that headache sufferers experience a variety of symptoms across headache attacks; however, the question is still whether these different attacks mirror the muscle-contraction–migraine dichotomy as laid down by the traditional diagnostic system. This is an extremely important empirical issue because most physicians, although recognizing symptom overlap as a common phenomenon in chronic patients, interpret symptom overlap as reflecting the presence of more than one *type* of headache in their patients:

> Many patients, especially those who have had chronic headache for years, have more than one type of headache which may occur as separate events but are more likely to blur into one another. It is quite common to see one who has had migraine for years develop a daily constant headache in middle age. This daily persistent headache may be punctuated by vascular, migraine-like attacks. Others may have distinct and separate attacks of migraine and muscle contraction head-

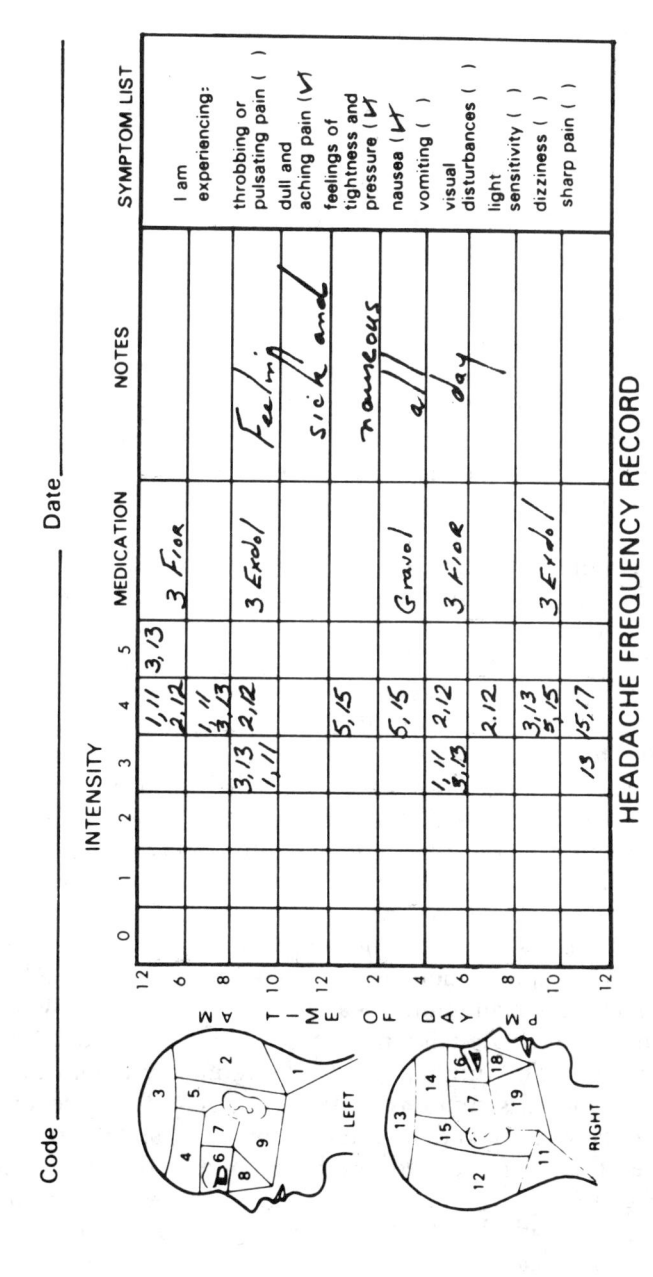

Figure 4.2 Sample headache frequency record used in the daily monitoring of headache activity.

ache. The term "mixed headache" is used to describe these combinations of headaches. Because of the frequent occurrence of several types of headache in the same person, a variety of medications may be necessary to control the symptoms. (Kunkel, 1979, p. 122)

The first study with the headache frequency record involved fifty-six chronic headache patients who had been diagnosed by neurologists as suffering from migraine, muscle-contraction, or combined migraine/muscle-contraction headache (Bakal & Kaganov, 1977). All neurologists who made the diagnoses followed the standard diagnostic scheme. The patients monitored their headache activity on a daily basis for a two-week period and were required to place the completed card in the mail at the end of each day. In order to represent the pain locations associated with muscle-contraction and migraine headaches, the eighteen locations on the card were reduced to five basic head regions. Migraine headache was represented by unilateral pain in the region of the eye and unilateral pain from the forehead. Bilateral pain from the neck, from the back/top of the head, and from the forehead were regions chosen to reflect the pain of muscle-contraction headache. A fifth area was included for bilateral pain from the eyes and sides of the head.

The degree of involvement of the various areas across headache attacks during the self-observation period was expressed as a proportion based on the number of headache hours an area was affected relative to the total number of hours of head pain experienced. The method of scoring made it possible to quantify with precision the degree to which the three diagnostic groups experienced muscle-contraction and migraine pain locations within and across their headache attacks. The results of the group comparisons on the frequency and intensity measures are presented in Figure 4.3. Contrary to traditional expectations, the three diagnostic groups were virtually identical in terms of the proportion of headache attacks associated with muscle-contraction and migraine head pain locations. This was also true of their average rated intensities of pain associated with the different locations. The original headache frequency record did not contain the associated symptoms section (Figure 4.2). However, the fifty-six patients were asked to indicate on a separate assessment form whether they experienced throbbing and/or dull and aching pain, visual disturbances, nausea/vomiting, and whether they had a family history of headache. Forty percent of migraine and muscle-contraction patients had throbbing headaches. Also, 52 percent of the patients from each group reported associated visual disturbances.

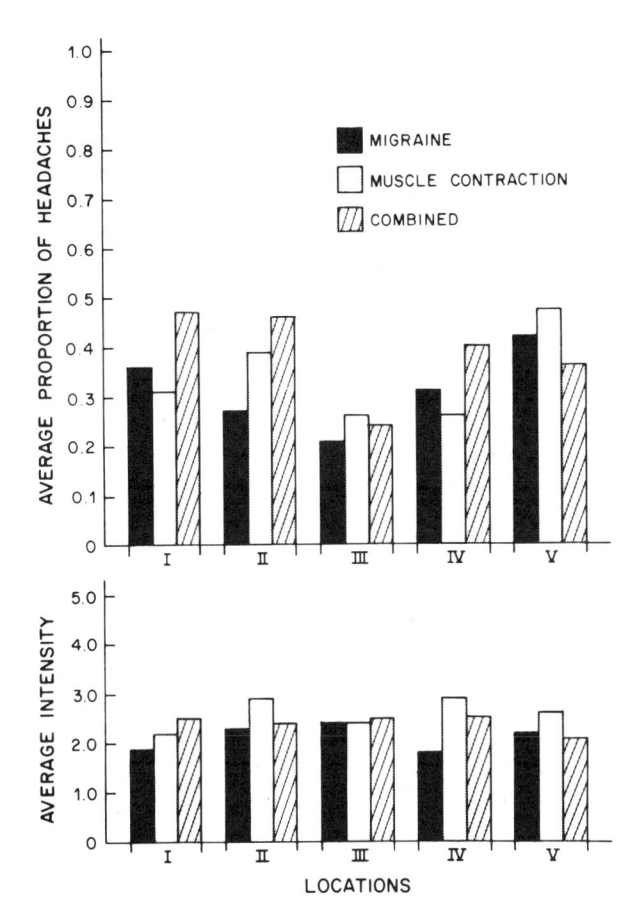

Figure 4.3 Proportions of headaches and pain intensities at specific locations. I: neck; II: forehead; III: side of head, eye (unilateral); IV: forehead (unilateral); V: sides of head, eyes. Intensity of pain reported at each location (Bakal & Kaganov, 1977). Copyright © 1977 by the American Association for the Study of Headache. Reprinted by permission of the publisher.

Forty-four percent of migraine patients and 48 percent of muscle-contraction patients had a family history of headache. Only one symptom differentiated the two diagnostic groups. Nausea and vomiting occurred more often in migraine patients (72 percent) than in muscle-contraction headache patients (36 percent).

Overall, muscle-contraction and migraine headache patients were found to be equally familiar with head pain locations and symptoms thought to be diagnostic of each group. The symptom similarities were not superficial since the proportions of headache attacks associated with specific locations were similar for both categories of headache patients. The results were not due to the migraine patients simply experiencing periodic muscle-contraction headaches since the locations, although varying from attack to attack, showed no tendency to fall into distinct migraine and muscle-contraction symptom clusters. It is important to re-emphasize that these observations do not mean that all headache sufferers are the same in terms of their pain locations and associated symptoms. On the contrary, each patient examined in this study exhibited a degree of uniqueness with respect to his or her headache activity. At the same time, however, the data suggest that the idiosyncratic nature of each patient's headache disorder is not adequately captured by the traditional diagnostic system. Symptom "overlap" is not an isolated event; it is a major characteristic of these patients and its presence needs to be examined in the context of developing headache disorders.

Olesen (1978) has reported some clinical observations of migraine patients that are quite consistent with the self-observation data. Rather than ask patients to retrospectively describe their symptoms, Olesen observed and recorded his patients' symptoms during a period when they were having an actual migraine attack. After examining some 750 patients, Olesen was surprised to discover that very few patients manifested what would be considered a typical migraine profile. The traditional symptoms of throbbing pain, unilateral pain, and visual disturbances were as frequently absent as they were present in these patients. In addition, the presence of associated migraine symptoms (nausea, vomiting, diarrhea, visual disturbances) was not related either to the quality of pain (throbbing/pulsating) or to any particular head pain location. The only symptom that was present in more than 50 percent of Olesen's patients was nausea, a symptom that is handled just as easily by the severity model as it is by the traditional model.

There is a counter-argument to the studies indicating that pure cultures of migraine and muscle-contraction headaches do not exist in clinical populations. The argument is based on the source of the data contained in these studies, which is the patients themselves. Since these patients are by definition chronic headache sufferers, the suspicion is that they most likely have acquired a hodgepodge of symptom characteristics over the years that may now be masking their original headache disorder. This argument is usually reserved for migraine patients who exhibit concomitant muscle-contraction symptoms and is not invoked to explain muscle-contraction patients who exhibit concomitant migraine symptoms. Kunkel (1979) expressed this argument very well in the following statement:

> All of us dealing with the chronic headache patient would classify most of the headaches that we see as being of the mixed variety. This includes muscle contraction as well as depression and tension, and those with vascular features. Early in the patient's history, before he or she had had the headache for all those years, you might well have been able to separate out the distinct migraine attacks, which did not often have the muscle contraction component. (p. 126)

There are at least two ways to determine the accuracy of this statement: the first is to examine headache symptom configurations in children, and the second is to examine headache symptom configurations in the general population, at a stage before the disorder has become a chronic medical problem.

Headache Symptoms in Children

A surprising number of children and adolescents are familiar with headache. For example, Deubner (1977) reported that 78 percent of a sample of 205 ten-to-twelve-year-olds reported having experienced headache. Problem headache is also one of the most frequent clinical entities seen by pediatric neurologists. Jay and Tomasi (1981) examined the hospital records of a pediatric unit within a children's hospital and found that 22 percent of the referrals were for recurrent headache. Neurologists routinely assume that muscle-contraction and migraine headache syndromes are clearly discernible in children, even more so than the syndromes are discernible in adult headache sufferers. Very few studies available have systematically assessed headache symptom configurations in children. Most of the data available are secondhand in that the symptom characteristics were obtained from parent descriptions, school records, medical reports, and not from the children themselves.

The psychobiological processes that control headache in children is at the heart of understanding the processes that control headache in adults. Medical experts often imply that headache in children is a self-limiting disorder, occurring in response to some family crisis that when resolved leads to a disappearance of the disorder. And yet, anecdotal data indicate that headache is by no means self-limiting, that in many instances it continues to plague the child through adolescence and adulthood. What needs to be determined is whether children exhibit relatively homogeneous headache syndromes or whether their symptom characteristics mark the beginnings of the symptom characteristics seen in adult headache sufferers. A related issue is whether headache in children occurs in the context of relatively specific events, at least initially, and then with repeated attacks beings to exhibit the functionally autonomous pattern that was observed to characterize adult headache sufferers.

The best known and most exhaustive study of headache in children was conducted by Bille (1962). He studied headache incidence and headache symptom configurations in a sample of 8,993 school children between the ages of seven and fifteen. Each child in the study was given a headache questionnaire that was to be completed by his or her parents. Since Bille was interested only in the occurrence of migraine symptoms in children, the questionnaire contained only items thought to be diagnostic of migraine. The actual questions that the parents were asked to complete for their children were as follows:

> If your son/daughter suffers from headaches at present, or has had headaches when younger, are they or have they been accompanied by one or any of the following signs which could indicate *migraine*?
> (a) Does the headache occur in sudden attacks, and is it completely absent between these attacks?
> (b) Is the headache more intense on one side than on the other?
> (c) Is the headache sometimes accompanied by nausea or vomiting?
> (d) Is there sometimes a bright flickering light in front of the eyes, just before the headache begins?
> (e) Do any relatives (siblings, parents) suffer from headaches of the type described here (migraine)?

Bille found that 347 children (3.9 percent) met the criteria of having paroxysmal headache, as determined by their response to question (a) on the inventory, and two of the additional characteristics. Unfortunately, Bille ignored some potentially valuable observations of children who experienced headache but who did not possess at least three migraine characteristics. Over 50 percent of the remaining children experienced some type of headache that was simply classified as "nonmigrainous" in nature. In any case, Bille found that the number of children with migraine increased linearly with age. The most frequently experienced region of unilateral pain was the forehead (45 percent) and not the eye (18 percent) or the temple (8 percent), as is believed to be the case for adult headache sufferers. The majority of attacks were described as having their onset during or after school, and the children themselves listed schoolwork and watching television as being the most frequent triggers of their attacks. The attacks were also of shorter duration than is typical of adult headache sufferers, with the average duration being approximately three hours.

Deubner (1977) conducted an epidemiologic study of headache in 600 ten-to-twenty-year-olds. Each subject was visited at home and a migraine questionnaire was completed by the parent. In addition, a subsample of ninety-seven subjects was interviewed directly by a pediatric neurologist and classified as suffering from migraine or nonmigrainous headache. By both the questionnaire and the neurologist, migraine was defined as the presence of unilateral headache, nausea with or without vomiting, and the presence of one or more of the following neurologic symptoms: scotomata, scintillations, paresthesias, and anesthesias. (It is difficult to comprehend the rationale behind assuming that the presence of one or two headache symptoms is indicative of nonmigrainous headache, whereas the same two symptoms plus one more becomes migraine headache.) Based on the questionnaire data, 74 percent of the male respondents and 82 percent of the female respondents were observed to have experienced headache. Of those with headache, 15.5 percent of males and 22.1 percent of females had all three migraine symptoms present. Larger percentages were observed for the headache respondents who had one or two symptoms present. For example, 30 percent of males with headaches and 43 percent of females with headaches reported their pain to be one-sided. Thirty-five percent of each sex had nausea with headache. It is interesting to note that there was considerable disagreement between the parents' descriptions of their children's headache symptoms and the children's descriptions as related to the neurologist. For example, of seventy-nine children who reported to the neurologist that they had two or three symptoms of migraine, fifty-six parents disagreed with this. Six parents believed that their children had no headaches at all!

Joffe, Bakal, and Kaganov (in press) completed a self-observation study of children and adolescents with problem headache. Rather than rely on parental observations, the children themselves monitored their headache activity on a daily basis for a three-week period. The self-observation record was identical in nature to the one used in the study of adult headache sufferers, except for cosmetic modifications that were made to make the record more attractive to children. Self-observation data were obtained from forty-seven children with problem recurrent headaches. The children ranged in age from eight to seventeen years, and they all seemed capable of keeping a daily record of the location of their pain as well as the presence or absence of associated symptoms.

The head pain locations and symptoms experienced by the children showed no tendency to cluster into muscle-contraction and migraine headache categories, as expected within the traditional diagnostic system. However, the children did exhibit some interesting relationships between the severity of their disorder and the symptoms experienced. Severity was defined primarily in terms of the number of attacks experienced, hours of head pain, and number (rather than kind) of symptoms experienced. The three measures were found to be positively related, which suggested that as the disorder becomes more frequent in nature, it also begins to encompass more symptoms. There was no evidence to suggest that some of the children began their headache disorder with migraine and acquired muscle-contraction symptoms as a secondary reaction. Since this was a cross-sectional rather than a longitudinal study, such a possibility cannot be ruled out. However, it is equally possible that the children began their headache history with isolated muscle-contraction and/or migraine symptoms and later developed additional symptoms from both categories.

Joffe et al. also presented data that suggested that muscle-contraction and migraine headache symptoms develop concomitantly across the dimension of headache severity. A positive correlation was found between the number of muscle-contraction symptoms reported and the number of migraine symptoms reported, and both these measures correlated positively with the number of attacks experienced during the self-observation period. The pain location and symptom overlap observed in the adult patients was found to characterize children with problem headache as well. In fact, the children seemed to constitute a microcosm of what may be called the "headache universe." Unlike the adult patients, they showed much more variability in their headache characteristics (pain locations, duration of attacks, number of symptoms experienced), and these characteristics pointed strongly to the presence of a disorder which, if left untreated, may become progressively more severe and encompassing across time.

Another interesting observation made by Joffe et al. concerned the time of onset of the headache attacks that the children experienced. It was previously mentioned that adult chronic headache

One or More Kinds of Headache?

sufferers experience the majority of their attacks upon awakening or within a few hours upon awakening (Bakal, Demjen, & Kaganov, 1981). As shown in Figure 4.4, children with problem headache, when compared to adults, are distributed more evenly throughout the day in terms of the time at which their headaches typically begin. For the children, the time of onset measure was correlated with the number of head pain locations experienced, the number of symptoms experienced, and the average duration of their headache attacks. Children with the more severe headache activity experienced their attacks at an earlier time of the day than children with the less severe headache activity. The children with severe headache had progressed to a stage of chronicity that was quite comparable to that observed in the chronic adult patients, in that for both groups the disorder showed signs of operating relatively autonomously from the events that are known to trigger attacks in less severe headache sufferers.

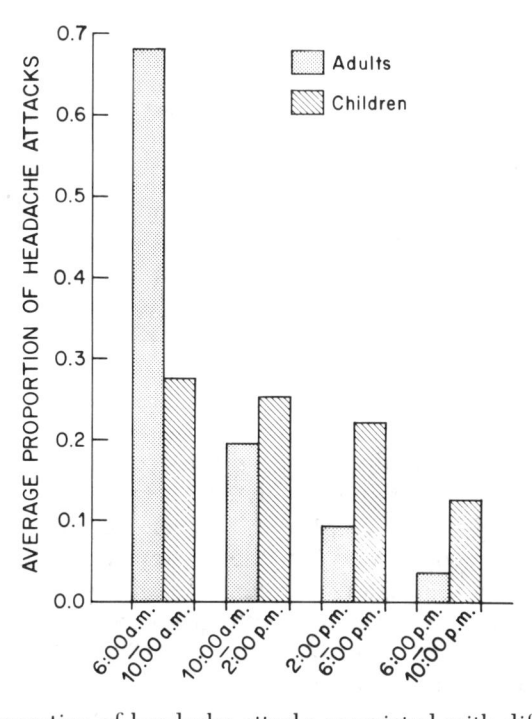

Figure 4.4 Proportion of headache attacks associated with different times of onset as observed by adult headache patients and children with problem headache (Joffe, Bakal, & Kaganov, in press).

Headache Symptoms in the Population

According to the National Migraine Foundation, the majority of headache sufferers in the population experience either muscle-contraction or migraine headache disorders, with the ratio being approximately three to one in favor of muscle-contraction symptoms. This is an assumption only and is without empirical support. In fact, the epidemiological literature is more consistent with a severity interpretation of headache symptoms than the traditional muscle-contraction–migraine dichotomy. As with chronic patients, symptom overlap is more often present than absent in headache sufferers within the population. The symptom configurations experienced by headache sufferers within the population often represent the beginnings of a disorder that progresses to chronicity; for this reason alone, it is important to understand how these symptoms cluster in the occasional or nonproblem headache sufferer.

The majority of existing epidemiological headache research comes not from North America but from Great Britain and Europe. The best known of these studies have been conducted by Waters (1973, 1974), and his findings have not supported the position that headache symptoms occur in the form of syndromes within the population. In his first study, Waters (1973) set out to determine the degree to which three of the major features of migraine (unilateral pain, prodromal warning, nausea) could be found to occur together within individuals in the general population. He administered a headache symptom questionnaire to a random sample of people with the instruction that they were to answer the items in reference to their headache activity during the previous year. Waters found no support for the presence of a migraine syndrome, as the three symptoms did not occur together much more frequently than would be expected by chance. Approximately one-third of the respondents who had any one of the symptoms did not have the other two, which indicated that the symptoms were not highly correlated with each other.

Waters (1974) has employed a second empirical argument to challenge those who believe in the existence of a distinct migraine syndrome. "True" migraine is often quoted as afflicting only a minority of headache sufferers, with guesstimates of its prevalence among headache sufferers ranging from 10 percent to 30 percent. However, Waters observed that almost all people who are familiar with headache are also familiar with at least one of the classical migraine symptoms. For example, of the respondents who had experienced headache during the previous year, 66 percent of the males and 71 percent of the females were familiar with one or more of the migraine symptoms. Equally high incidences of migraine symptoms have been reported by other epidemiological investigators (Green, 1977; Markush, Karp, Heyman, & O'Fallon, 1975; Ziegler, Hassanein, & Couch, 1977). Waters also had his subjects rate their headaches in terms of perceived severity (from very mild to almost unbearable) and found a positive relationship between the severity rating and the prevalence of the three migraine symptoms. Of the subjects who rated their headaches as mild, 30 percent had unilateral pain, 5 percent had a preheadache warning, and 20 percent experienced nausea. Of those with unbearable headaches, 55 percent had unilateral pain, 65 percent had a warning, and 75 percent experienced nausea. In short, the three migraine symptoms, although failing to occur in the form of a syndrome, increased concomitantly with headache severity. Waters proposed that migraine symptoms be viewed along a continuum of headache severity, with "mild headaches, usually unaccompained by the features of migraine, at one extreme and severe headaches, frequently accompanied by the features of migraine, at the other."

Waters' main theoretical concern was with migraine symptom configurations in the population, and he did not assess the prevalence of muscle-contraction symptoms in his subjects. Muscle-contraction symptoms have been neglected by most epidemiological researchers. An exception to this tendency is the research of Kaganov (1980). She devised a survey questionnaire that contains items indicative of both muscle-contraction and migraine symptoms. Another advantage of her questionnaire is that it does not force the respondents to describe headaches in terms of their "most typical" or "most severe" attacks. Instead, the fourteen symptom items are presented along a five-point continuum that allows the respondents to describe the full range of their headache experiences, from pain locations and symptoms that are rarely experienced to pain locations and symptoms that are always experienced. The questionnaire also contains an item that asks the respondents to indicate how often they consider their headaches to be a problem. This item is used to differentiate the occasional headache sufferer from the individual who experiences headache on a chronic basis.

The first study with the questionnaire (Bakal & Kaganov, 1979) compared symptom characteristics of college students and chronic headache patients. The purpose of the study was to determine the extent to which the expected symptom differences could be portrayed along a continuum of headache severity. All the respondents were initially classified into three groups: (1) those who never or seldom perceived their headaches to be a problem; (2) those who sometimes perceived their headaches to be a problem; and (3) those who often or always perceived their headaches to be a problem. The first group was comprised totally of students and the last group was comprised of chronic headache patients, with the exception of three students. The results indicated that the fourteen pain locations and symptoms assessed by the questionnaire were present to some extent in all three groups—the differences being quantitative rather than qualitative. A second analysis involved a comparison of the symptom frequencies experienced by patients who had been diagnosed as migraineurs with the symptom frequencies experienced by the other respondents. As shown in Figure 4.5, the migraine patients were not only familiar with all fourteen pain locations and symptoms, but they also reported experiencing these locations and symptoms more frequently than the other headache sufferers. These findings have been replicated in an independent study by Thompson, Haber, Figueroa, and Adams (1980).

The data contained in Figure 4.5 illustrate another significant finding of this study. Muscle-contraction headache symptoms such as neck pain, top of head pain, and tightness and pressure were experienced more frequently by migraineurs than several of the more traditional migraine symptoms such as throbbing pain, unilateral pain, and visual disturbances. Thus, the symptom data obtained in this study reinforce the physiological observations made in the previous chapter, which suggested that heightened muscle activity plays a significant role in the etiology and maintenance of severe headache disorders. The frequency data for the entire sample was subjected to a multiple step-wise regression analysis using problem as the dependent variable. This statistic represents a method of analyzing the collective and separate contributions of two or more independent variables to the variation of the dependent variable. Five symptoms each contributed to a significant separate proportion of the variance, and taken together these symptoms accounted for 57.3 percent of the total variance explained. Nausea accounted for 33 percent of the variance associated with problem headaches. The remaining symptoms and the additional variances accounted for were the following, in descending order: neck (13 percent), top of head (6.5 percent), tightness and pressure (2.8 percent), and forehead (2 percent). In summary, the variables that best accounted for the variance asso-

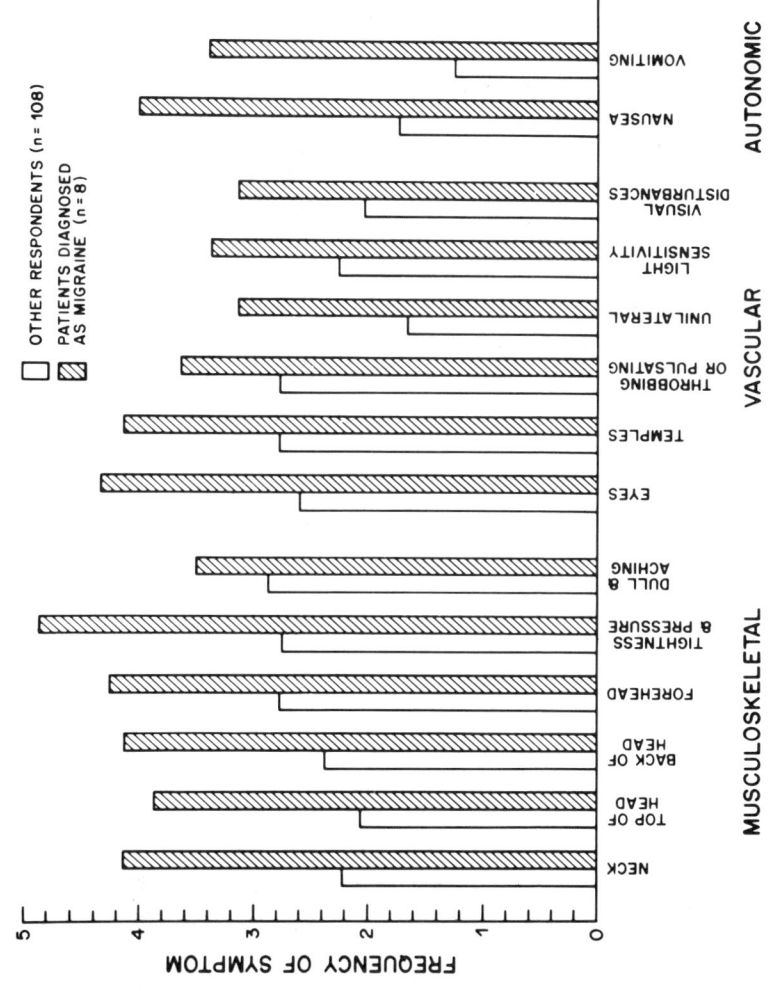

Figure 4.5 Frequencies of symptoms reported by the migraine patients and by the remaining respondents (Bakal & Kaganov, 1979). Copyright © 1979 by the American Association for the Study of Headache.

ciated with problem headaches were nausea and musculoskeletal symptoms commonly associated with muscle-contraction headache.

The next application of the Kaganov questionnaire explored the configuration of muscle-contraction and migraine headache symptoms in the general population (Kaganov, Bakal, & Dunn, 1981). Questionnaires were obtained from 785 randomly selected households, and it was demonstrated that all fourteen pain locations and symptoms were present to some extent across the problem headache dimension. Thirteen of the fourteen symptoms showed a positive relationship between their frequency of occurrence and the extent to which headaches were perceived to be a problem. Similar symptom distributions were observed to occur for males and females. The population frequency data across the fourteen symptoms for females and males are presented in Figure 4.6. Although females (including those as young as thirteen years of age) were observed to experience all symptoms more frequently than males, the differences were not that notable. What was impressive is that the patterns of frequencies

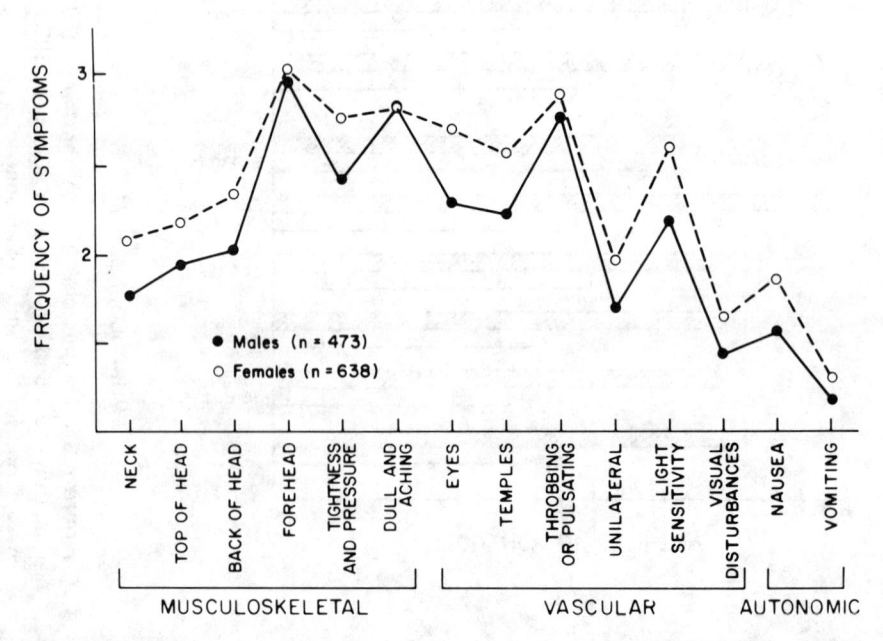

Figure 4.6 Frequencies of headache symptoms reported to be present across headache attacks (Kaganov, Bakal, & Dunn, 1981). Copyright © 1981 by the American Association for the Study of Headache. Reprinted by permission of the publisher.

across the two sexes were identical. The symptoms that were experienced the most and the least frequently by the two groups were virtually the same. The symptoms associated with problem headache in the female were no different from the symptoms associated with problem headache in the male; the female simply was afflicted slightly more often.

Problem headache was associated with a shift from musculoskeletal symptom dominance to vascular symptom dominance across the problem headache dimension. As shown in Figure 4.7, individuals who never or seldom viewed headache as a problem experienced musculoskeletal symptoms more frequently than they experienced vascular symptoms, while individuals who often or always considered headache to be a problem experienced vascular symptoms more frequently than musculoskeletal symptoms. Both categories of symptoms increased with problem headache, but vascular symptoms increased at a more rapid rate. The shift in symptom dominance was not due to a decrease in the involvement of musculoskeletal symptoms with more problematic headaches. Muscle-contraction symptoms also increased across the problem dimension but to a lesser extent than vascular symptoms. Also there was no evidence that the various symptoms clustered in accordance with the diagnostic categories of muscle-contraction and migraine headaches. Rather, both types of symptoms were positively related in that an increase in the number of migraine symptoms experienced was matched by an increase in the number of muscle-contraction symptoms experienced. In addition, both types of symptoms also correlated positively with the extent to which headaches were perceived to be a problem and with headache frequency. These data suggest that increasingly severe and frequent headache attacks are accompanied by the increasing involvement of both migraine and muscle-contraction headache symptoms, and not by a qualitative change in the types of symptoms experienced.

In summary, there are considerable data that support the utility of viewing headache symptoms along a continuum of severity. There is little evidence that the symptoms of muscle-contraction and migraine headaches occur in the form of two distinct clusters. On the contrary, muscle-contraction symptoms were observed to occur concomitantly with vascular and autonomic symptoms in clinical patients, in children with problem headache, and in occasional headache sufferers. The fact that headache sufferers experience some configuration of both musculoskeletal and vascular symptoms suggests that the respective physiological systems influence and are

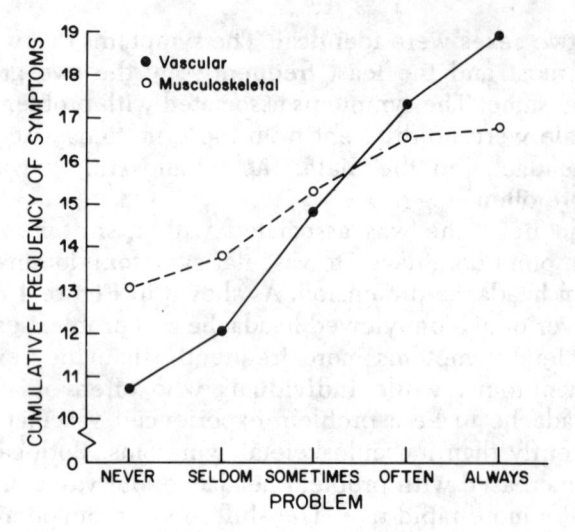

Figure 4.7 Comparison of musculoskeletal symptoms with vascular symptoms across the problem headache dimension (Kaganov, Bakal, & Dunn, 1981). Copyright © 1981 by the American Association for the Study of Headache. Reprinted by permission of the publisher.

influenced by each other's presence. These data support the hypothesis that similar psychobiological processes underlie all headache sufferers, ranging from the person who experiences only the occasional mild headache to the chronic patient who experiences severe recurrent headache attacks. This does not mean that the physiological mechanisms underlying all headaches are the same, but rather that similar psychobiological processes initiate the disorder, with the processes becoming more involved as the disorder increases in severity. From this perspective, chronic headache represents one end of a severity continuum rather than a unique disease process distinct from the processes controlling nonproblem headache.

5
Clinical and Theoretical Concerns

In previous chapters, arguments and supporting data were presented for viewing chronic headache from a psychobiological or severity perspective. It should now be apparent to the reader that the new perspective does not constitute a radical departure from existing knowledge of headache per se. In fact, much of the empirical support for the model was based on psychological, physiological, and symptom data that often have been used by traditionalists to support their theoretical position. At the same time, however, the psychobiological approach demands a shift to more holistic constructs, and in doing so it provides a conceptual framework for integrating the various aspects of headache research within a unitary framework. Several theoretical issues need to be discussed before the full potential of the model can be realized, and this represents the objective behind this chapter. Some of the issues are at the heart of medical diagnosis of headache, whereas others deal with the problems faced by patients themselves in comprehending the personal significance of the severity model.

Dimension Versus Syndrome

Viewing headache symptoms along a continuum of severity has major implications for clinicians who are accustomed to understanding symptoms as being indicative of headaches with different etiologies.

Of course, the severity model cannot account for organic headache, but organic headache is a low-probability event. Just as the severity model cannot handle headaches that are due to organic factors, the medical model cannot handle headaches that are due to psychobiological factors. Physicians are trained extensively in diagnosis, and it is understandable that they might have some difficulty in accepting the notion of a symptom continuum.

Some medical specialists believe that viewing headache symptoms along a severity continuum implies that all headaches are the same. Arnold Friedman (cited in Kunkel, 1979) expressed his concern, as well as that of many of his medical colleagues, as follows:

> I also am interested in the comments on ... the idea that headaches should be lumped together, very much as Gertrude Stein said "a rose is a rose is a rose." I don't agree that you can say that "a headache is a headache" unless you want to revert back to about 1893. I do not think that you can ignore the tremendous amount of experimental work, clinical work, and expertise of men such as Harold Wolff and the Cornell group (and many others) indicating that there are indeed differences in various types of headache. (p. 126)

The severity model does not state that one headache is the same as the next headache. It states that similar psychobiological processes, and not necessarily symptoms, underlie all headache sufferers. In effect, the model allows for dynamic interplay between symptoms in the development of chronic headache disorders. If anything, "lumping" seems more likely to occur with a system that forces the majority of patients with diverse symptom configurations into one of two diagnostic categories. There is also little evidence that the system has provided physicians with an effective means of differentially treating headache disorders. The issue of medical treatment is examined later in this chapter.

Physicians often defend the traditional diagnostic system on the grounds that it provides them with some knowledge of the origins and future course of different headache disorders. There is little evidence that this is the case. However, a thorny issue that still remains with respect to classification is this: if symptom differences are not indicative of qualitatively different headache disorders, then what are symptom differences indicative of? Some patients experience unilateral pain while other patients do not. Some patients experience headache attacks that are highly localized, while other patients experience pain that is diffuse in nature. Even in patients who are equated in terms of subjective severity of the pain experienced, there are often marked symptom differences. For example, migraine and cluster headache attacks are equally painful but are noticeably different in their symptomatologies. Migraine attacks are less frequent, do not appear in clusters, have a longer duration, have a throbbing quality, and are associated with nausea and vomiting. With migraine and cluster headaches, we have some of the strongest evidence for distinct kinds of symptom configurations. However, the distinction may exist mainly at the symptom level and not at the etiologic level. That is, migraine and cluster may appear on the surface to represent two distinct types of headache disorders, but both may be under the control of similar psychobiological processes. The symptom differences may represent structural-anatomical differences between the two types of patients more than they do etiologic differences. Cluster headache can be understood along the same lines as muscle-contraction and migraine headaches. It is interesting in this regard that cluster headache can increase in severity to the point that it occurs in the complete absence of remission periods. Also these patients are able to learn to regulate their attacks by using the same self-control procedures that are taught to muscle-contraction and migraine headache sufferers.

Another critical symptom characteristic that physicians and patients alike use in their argument that migraine is no "ordinary" headache is the presence of preheadache or prodromal symptoms. Prodromal symptoms, such as visual disturbances, are also at the basis of the distinction between classical migraine and common migraine. Most patients who experience preheadache symptoms do not experience these symptoms with a high degree of distinctiveness. For example, visual symptoms are usually described in terms of slight blurring or other minor distortions. Only a few patients experience zigzag patterns, blind spots, and flashing lights. These symptoms cannot be detected in most patients who are diagnosed and treated as migraineurs. Possibly it is this fact that makes diagnosticians skeptical of questionnaires that simply ask respondents to report the presence or absence of "visual disturbances" and that do not attempt to assess the quality of the disturbances. Under such a broad and loose definition, almost all headache sufferers will appear to have these symptoms. This constitutes a valid criticism, but at the same time it does not invalidate the severity model. Marked visual disturbances represent interesting neurophysiological phenomena that need to be explained, but there is no evidence to date that suggests that their presence constitutes proof of a unique headache syndrome. It is still reasonable to assume that the processes controlling headaches in these individuals are no different than the processes controlling headaches that are not preceded by such dramatic symptoms.

Each headache sufferer is in some respects a unique individual, not only in terms of his or her particular symptom configurations but also in terms of thoughts and feelings that accompany the disorder. In time it may be possible to reduce the various symptom configurations to a finite number of categories. However, such an accomplishment would not necessarily mean that different headache disorders had been identified, with each disorder having a different etiology.

The psychobiological model does not demand that physicians abandon their approach to headache diagnosis. A working relationship between the medical model and the psychobiological model in terms of patient assessment can be accomplished by substituting the word *description* for the word *diagnosis*. Diagnosis is after all a more appropriate approach when the disorder at issue is under the control of some biological condition. Even most headache experts recognize that this is not the case with muscle-contraction and migraine headaches. For example, Diamond and Dalessio (1978) stated that "severe headache is only infrequently caused by organic disease ... it may be inferred that for the most part headache represents an inability of the individual to deal in some measure with the uncertainties of life—that it is a symptom of wrong pace or wrong direction rather than a structural disease of the nervous system." Given that headache involves all aspects of human functioning, it seems reasonable to adopt an approach that permits the description of all components of the headache syndrome. Using the labels "muscle-contraction" and "migraine" in a descriptive rather than in a diagnostic fashion has the advantage of facilitating a conceptual awareness of the dynamic interplay that takes place between the various systems that make up the chronic headache patient. For example, the concomitant presence of muscle-contraction and migraine symptoms suggests a shared etiological mechanism for both categories of symptoms, which is quite different from the traditional diagnostic view that such a phenomenon reflects two different kinds of headache disorder in the same patient. A descriptive approach to classification also avoids the implicit paradox that migraine is a basic biochemical disorder on the one hand, and is due to stress or problems of living on the other hand. A descriptive analysis allows not only for the interplay of behaviors at one level of abstraction (e.g., physiological) but also for the interplay of behaviors from different levels of abstraction (psychological, physiological, biochemical).

The Role of Drugs in Headache Management

The psychobiological model of headache demands a holistic approach not only to headache assessment but also to headache treatment. The most frequently used method of headache management is medication, and medication has as its foundation a biomedical model of headache. Since medication is the principal therapeutic resource that physicians use in their daily practice of dealing with chronic headache sufferers, they are likely to be quite concerned with the proposal that their patients' headache disorders cannot be controlled with medication alone. This section takes a critical look at various drugs that are currently used to control headache. The discussion does not constitute a critique of drug use per se, but rather a critique of current thinking behind drug use. Drugs have a useful role to play in the management of headache disorders, but the general understanding of what can be expected with drugs needs to be altered. Drugs alone cannot be expected to regulate psychobiological disorders. The theory and application of drugs with psychobiological disorders requires an approach different from that underlying the use of drugs associated with biomedical disorders.

Drugs in Use for Controlling Muscle-Contraction Headache

Muscle-contraction headache is generally treated with prescription analgesics in the form of APC and APC-like drugs. An APC drug contains aspirin in combination with phenacetin and caffeine. Phenacetin is an analgesic with properties very similar to those found in salicylate. Caffeine is regularly included in these drugs because it also has analgesic properties. Acetaminophen and propoxyphene are additional analgesic substances that are found in some APC-like drugs. It is generally recognized that the various combinations of these substances are chosen primarily for commercial exploitation rather than for known therapeutic effects. Although containing different substances, trade name compounds such as Darvon, Tylenol, and Phrenelin have not been demonstrated to be differentially effective in controlling muscle-contraction headache, and in many instances they have not even been found to be more effective than placebos (Evans, 1974). A popular prescription analgesic is Fiorinal, which is a mixture of aspirin, phenacetin, caffeine, and butabital (a barbiturate). Although advertised as the "specializer" for muscle-contraction headache, its pain reduction qualities have been grossly overstated. In fact, no known analgesic reliably and effectively controls chronic muscle-contraction headache.

Antianxiety drugs, or anxiolytics, were widely used to control muscle-contraction symptoms for a period, but the use of such compounds has decreased following public outcry over the general abuse of these drugs. The most widely used anxiolytics for headache are chlordiazepoxide (Librium) and diazepam (Valium). Although not analgesics per se, both drugs are capable of attenuating the distress that accompanies headache attack (Greenblatt & Shader, 1974). Both drugs also are believed to have muscle relaxant properties. Although these drugs may attenuate the pain of a headache patient, the patient learns nothing of the conditions controlling the disorder. Consequently, the frequency of attacks remains unaltered, and the patient may develop a dependency on the drug as well as hyperalgesia such that he or she hurts more with the drug present than with the drug absent (Halpern, 1978). A factor contributing to the decreased use of anxiolytics is traceable to a phenomenon occurring in the general population. Anxiety is being rivalled by depression as the psychological disorder experienced most frequently by the populace and, given the prevalence of both depression and muscle-contraction headaches, it is not surprising to find clinicians believing that depression, and not anxiety, is the principal cause of muscle-contraction headaches.

A frequently prescribed antidepressant for headache is amitriptyline chloride (Elavil). There is some empirical support for using it as a prophylactic for chronic headache, but there is also evidence that amitriptyline's effectiveness is not due to antidepressant properties per se. Couch and Hassanein (1979) performed a double-blind comparison of amitriptyline and placebo in which all patients were initially given placebo for a four-week baseline period and then were randomly assigned to therapy with amitriptyline or placebo for another four to eight weeks. Subjects were given up to four 25-mg tablets of amitriptyline hydrochloride or identical placebo per day. The response to therapy was evaluated by comparing improvement from the last week of the baseline period to the last week of the treatment period. The dependent variable consisted of a severity score reflecting the weighted average of frequency, duration, and degree of disability associated with headache attacks. Of the patients who received amitriptyline, 55 percent showed a reduction of at least 50 percent in their severity scores. It is interesting that 50 percent reductions in severity scores also occurred in 34 percent of the pa-

Clinical and Theoretical Concerns

tients who received placebos. Depression was assessed by the use of depression rating scales. Taking the measures of severity and depression together, Couch and Hassanein found that the patients who responded best to amitriptyline were those who were *nondepressed* with severe headache, followed by those who were depressed with mild headache. Depressed patients with severe headache experienced no relief.

Couch and Hassanein concluded that the observed effectiveness of amitriptyline was not likely due to its antidepressant effects but was possibly due to the drug's ability to directly alter the neurophysiochemical mechanisms associated with head pain. An equally plausible hypothesis is that amitriptyline altered the *psychobiological susceptibility* of these patients to headache attacks. This susceptibility is comprised of cognitive, affective, sensory, and physiochemical variables, and amitriptyline may have led to nonspecific changes in all of these variables. Also, the observation that nondepressed patients with severe headache did not respond to drug therapy may have been due to the fact that these patients were experiencing considerable distress with their headache attacks. (Recall from the discussion in Chapter 2 that measures of depression actually may reflect the psychological distress that accompanies the chronic headache syndrome.) Patients who scored high on depression in this study may simply have been experiencing too much distress to have responded to amitriptyline administration alone.

Migraine Medication

The pharmacological treatment of migraine headache is generally assumed to be based on a much more solid rationale than the drug treatment of muscle-contraction headache. Because of the presumed vascular sequence of migraine, i.e., vasoconstriction during the prodrome followed by vasodilation during the headache, there are a number of drugs available for regulating and/or altering these vascular events. Methysergide maleate (Sansert) was the first antimigraine drug to be used as a prophylactic. Methysergide is believed to exert its prophylactic action by potentiating the effect of other vasoconstrictor agents such as norepinephrine (Dalessio, 1980b). Propranolol (Inderol) is a second prophylactic agent in common use, and it is hypothesized to prevent the onset of vasodilation by blocking the action of the beta-adrenergic receptors located in the smooth muscle walls of the arterioles. Another prophylactic compound is clonidine hydrochloride (Catapres), which, although considered to be primarily an antihypertensive compound, is now being used to prevent headache.

Are prophylactic compounds effective in preventing headache associated with migraine symptoms? In fact, such compounds may not be that effective, at least to the degree of being more effective than drugs that do not have specific vasoactive properties. Couch and Hassanein (1979) examined the existing literature on prophylactics with the specific aim of determining the percentage of patients who, in the various studies of prophylactic compounds, showed a reduction of at least 50 percent in their post-treatment headache activity. Using this criterion, they found that in eight studies involving methysergide the average patient improvement rate was 58.3 percent, a figure that is comparable to the improvement rate of 55 percent obtained with antidepressant medication. In five studies involving propranolol, 51.6 percent of the total number of patients showed improvement, while in six studies using clondine hydrochloride, 40.9 percent of the patients showed improvement. Different drugs with different physiochemical effects seem to produce roughly equivalent therapeutic effects—approximately 50 percent of patients show reductions in headache activity following their administration.

The main compound for controlling the pain of an actual migraine attack is ergotamine tartrate. Ergotamine's therapeutic action is believed to result from its ability to produce a powerful and a prolonged vasoconstriction of the extracranial vasculature (Dalessio, 1980b). Several commercial ergotamine compounds are in use, some of which contain only ergotamine (Gynergen) while others contain ergotamine in combination with one or more APC compounds. For example, Cafergot contains ergotamine and caffeine, while Wigraine contains ergotamine, caffeine, phenacetin, and belladonna. Although ergotamine drugs are often cited as being extremely effective in the control of migraine pain, this is simply not the case. The majority of patients referred to our clinic have at one time or another received a regimen of ergotamine therapy and none have experienced lasting relief. Olesen, Aebelholdt, and Veilis (1979) also presented a pessimistic view of the clinical usefulness of ergotamine. After clinically examining some 750 migraine patients, they concluded that ergotamine had little therapeutic value and that in some patients ergotamine seemed to *cause* rather than *prevent* the pain of migraine. The latter phenomenon is called *ergotamine-induced headache* and is suspected to result from a chronic state of vasoconstriction that develops from the prolonged use of ergotamine drugs.

The ergotamine headache was described by Andersson (1975) as follows:

> The headache was characteristically present all day. Patients awakened with pain often localized in the neck. This then spread to the temples and forehead. More than half the patients had more pronounced headache in the area where they had pain during attacks of migraine. The headache was uncomfortable, heavy and oppressive, and differed in intensity from day to day and throughout the day. Exacerbations of pain occurred among migraineurs and non-migraineurs, often leading to nausea and vomiting. These exacerbations were difficult to distinguish from true migraine attacks. They were also not easily distinguished from interval headache, because patients were never headache free. (p. 118)

Andersson's description of the ergotamine headache is virtually identical in terms of symptom characteristics to the syndrome that was previously described as characterizing chronic headache sufferers in general. It is inaccurate to attribute this condition to ergotamine alone given that the same condition can be detected in patients who have never taken ergotamine or who are no longer using ergotamine.

A general problem with all the drug-outcome literature is that empirical support exists for almost any compound in use for controlling headache disorders. However, it is questionable whether the various compounds have differential effectiveness. Most outcome studies are based on a comparison of a particular compound with a placebo. Seldom do these studies compare one drug compound with another drug compound. When this step is taken, the results are not supportive of a drug-specificity explanation. For example, Hakkarainen, Quiding, and Stockman (1980) compared the effectiveness of a mild analgesic (propoxyphene) with that of ergotamine for controlling acute migraine attacks. The comparison was made in a double-blind crossover study of twenty-five female patients. The analgesic was found to be as effective as ergotamine, and the analgesic was also associated with a reduced incidence of nausea and vomiting. Drug use patterns seem to mirror a severity position more than a specificity position. Chronic headache sufferers often report beginning their medication history with nonprescription analgesics and then in time move on to prescription analgesics before graduating to ergotamine compounds. Once ergotamine compounds become ineffective, they may again experience temporary relief from mild analgesics. Olesen et al. (1979) reported good short-term effects in treating migraine patients who no longer responded to ergotamine with a drug mixture based on a mild analgesic, a tranquilizer, and a substance designed to reduce nausea and vomiting. They reported that their particular pharmaceutical mixture was "67 percent effective in making migraine patients headache free within a few hours of administration." It appears that any new drug or change in drug regimen is capable of producing short-term relief. The problem is that drugs are generally not effective in the long run.

Evidence indicating that drugs are not effective in the long run comes from a survey study by Parnell and Cooperstock (1979). They mailed a drug use questionnaire to 1500 migraine sufferers and asked the respondents to indicate how effective they had found various drugs to be in controlling their headache attacks. Analgesics were rated as excellent by 23 percent of the respondents who used analgesics. Only 19.7 percent and 27.2 percent of the respondents who used prophylactics and ergotamine drugs rated these compounds as excellent. The rated effectiveness of tranquilizers and mood elevators was even worse, with 12.4 percent of the respondents rating these substances as excellent. Much larger percentages of the respondents rated the compounds as being "fair" in terms of effectiveness, but it may be a mistake to interpret this rating as support for drug effectiveness. Patients will often use the descriptor "fair" when they feel that the pain would have been worse had they not taken the drug. Virtually all our patients take medication with clocklike regularity even though their self-observation records show no change in the degree or duration of pain experienced following drug consumption. However, they all insist that the pain would be much worse without the medication.

Drugs and Headache-Related Behavior

The confusion surrounding the use of drugs to control headache is largely due to a misunderstanding of what can be expected from drugs. If, as proposed earlier, the various components of headache, including the psychological, physiological, and biochemical, are viewed as interacting *behaviors,* then it should be apparent that drugs alone cannot be expected to produce significant therapeutic changes. The complexities associated with predicting the behavioral effects of psychoactive drugs are now known to be enormous (Bakal, 1979), and the same can be said with respect to headache medications. It is necessary to understand not only the drug-produced changes in physiochemistry but also how these changes influence and are influenced by other components of the headache syndrome. A headache is a complex behavior and drugs do not create new behavior; they only influence existing behavior.

Drug researchers have attempted to rule out drug-behavior interactions by examining drug effects within the framework of double-blind research designs. In this situation, neither the experimenter nor the patient knows the nature of the compound being administered at any particular session. However, not informing a patient as to what he or she has ingested does not rule out cognitive variables but rather creates a kind of guessing game in which the patient is not certain whether he or she *should* or *should not* feel better. It is interesting that clinical studies of drugs that have failed to use double-blind procedures usually report success rates four-to-five times in excess of studies that have used double-blind procedures. The use of double-blind studies reflects the medical belief that any therapeutic change that is not due to biochemical alteration per se is due to placebo effects, and placebo effects have always had negative connotations in medicine. Although most physicians recognize the power of placebos, they still continue to view placebo-related effects as being *independent* from drug-produced effects. Prescriptions for minor analgesics and tranquilizers often are made on the grounds that such substances will make the patient "feel better if he or she has something to swallow." However, the same reasoning is seldom applied when the prescriptions involve more powerful compounds such as the ergotamine-based drugs.

According to Shapiro and Morris (1978), the placebo effect is the main reason why many forms of primitive treatment techniques used throughout the history of medicine were effective:

> Psychological factors, always important in medicine, were recognized as early as the period of Hippocrates. Galen estimated that 60 percent of patients had symptoms of emotional rather than physical origin. This figure is close to the contemporary estimate of 50 to 80 percent. Despite Galen's and Hippocrates' acumen, few if any of the drugs used by the physicians of their day caused pharmacologically induced therapeutic change. Treatment was primitive, unscientific, largely ineffective, and often shocking and dangerous....
>
> Patients took almost every known organic and inorganic substance—crocodile dung, teeth of swine, hooves of asses, spermatic fluid of frogs, eunuch fat, fly specks, lozenges of dried vipers, powder of precious stones, bricks, furs, feathers, hair, human perspiration, oil of ants, earthworms, wolves, spiders, moss scraped from the skull of a victim of violent death, and so on. Blood from every animal was pre-

pared and administered in every way and was used to treat every conceivable symptom and disease. Almost all human and animal excretions were used.

Some famous treatments used for centuries include the Royal Touch, Egyptian mummy, unicorn horn, bezoar stone, and mandrake. Theriac contained 37 to 63 ingredients; mattiolo contained 230 ingredients and required several months to concoct. Galen's elaborate pharmacopoeia, all worthless, contained 820 substances. Medical reasoning was primitive: Lung of fox, a long-winded animal, was given to consumptives. Fat of bear, a hirsute animal, was prescribed for baldness. Mistletoe, a plant that grows on the oak that cannot fall, was specific for the falling sickness.... A wound was treated by sympathetic powder that was applied to the inflicting implement. Throughout medical history patients were purged, puked, poisoned, punctured, cut, cupped, blistered, bled, leached, heated, frozen, sweated, and shocked.... Useful drugs or procedures were applied infrequently and were usually forgotten by succeeding generations. For thousands of years physicians prescribed what we now know were useless and often dangerous medications. This would have been impossible were it not for the fact that physicians did help their patients.

Today we know that the effectiveness of these procedures and medications was due to psychological factors often referred to as the placebo effect. Since almost all medications until recently were placebos, the history of medical treatment can be characterized largely as the history of the placebo effect. (p. 370)

In modern times, the placebo effect remains an important component of drug action and drug therapy. After reviewing fifteen studies, Beecher (1959) concluded that placebo medication successfully reduced pain in approximately 35 percent of the patients studied. Beecher also found the placebo to be more effective in relieving pain of clinical origin than pain of experimental origin. He also found morphine to be more effective in alleviating clinical pain than experimental pain:

Great wounds with great significance and presumably great reaction are made painless by small doses of morphine, whereas fleeting experimental pains with no serious significance are not blocked by morphine. The difference here in the two situations would seem to be in difference of significance of the two wounds. Morphine acts on significant pain, not on the other. (p. 164)

In a later article, Beecher (1975) proposed a "new principle of drug action," which is that some drugs are only effective in the presence of an appropriate mental state. An experience with a patient from our behavioral management program can be used to illustrate the importance of this principle. Prior to beginning the program, the patient would periodically admit herself, during a severe attack, to the emergency unit of a local hospital in order to receive an injection of morphine. The injection often made her nauseous and had little effect on the pain. Following training in self-management, she still had severe recurrent headaches and she still sought periodic relief at the hospital. However, the patient discovered that by "working with" the morphine injection (i.e., trying to relax), its therapeutic effects were almost immediate.

Evans (1974) reported some interesting observations that have a bearing on a psychobiological approach to pharmacology. He reviewed placebo analgesic studies with clinical pain that were conducted subsequent to Beecher's (1959) review. He found, similar to Beecher, that an average of 36 percent of patients achieve significant relief from pain after ingesting a placebo. He also found that the effectiveness of a placebo, when compared to a standard dose of a specific analgesic drug administered double-blind, is *constant*. That is, the effectiveness of the placebo is directly proportional to the apparent effectiveness of the active analgesic agent. To illustrate, the efficacy of placebo compared to morphine was .56, i.e., the placebo was 56 percent as effective as morphine. The index of placebo efficacy for aspirin was the same for both aspirin (.54) and intermediate strength Darvon (.56). "Thus, it appears that when the responsible physician knows that a powerful analgesic agent is being used (e.g., morphine), a *strong* placebo effect is obtained in a double-blind administration. If, however, it is assumed that the analgesic is less effective (e.g., aspirin), a much smaller placebo effect is obtained, even though it is still proportionately about half as effective as the actual analgesic."

Attempting to separate out placebo effects from drug effects creates the illusion that these are independent events, whereas in all likelihood they are not. When associated with improvement, placebo administration and drug administration most likely achieve their effects through the alteration of common physiological mechanisms. Such mechanisms are not recognized within the present connotation of the term *placebo effect*. Placebo effects do not reside within the environment, within enthusiastic physicians, or within large and colorful drug capsules (Shapiro & Morris, 1978). Although situational factors may facilitate the placebo effect, the effect itself resides within the patient. Patients possess the internal resources that determine not only whether or not a placebo capsule has a positive effect but also whether or not an active drug substance has a positive effect.

Headache sufferers seldom recognize that they have a major role to play in drug therapy and, if anything, they feel that it is the responsibility of their physician and the drug to alleviate their headache disorder. The dependency on medication prevents them from even considering the possibility that they might be able to gain control over their symptoms. The following case study, provided by Levendusky and Pankratz (1975), illustrates this phenomenon:

> Mr. X was a 65-year-old retired army officer with a history that included significant military achievement, a productive teaching and research career, and numerous social accomplishments. Medically, the patient had had frequent abdominal operations for gallstones, postoperative adhesions, and bowel obstructions. At the time of his voluntary hospitalization, he was complaining of continued abdominal pain, loss of weight, and social withdrawal.
>
> A mental status exam revealed an oriented, intact man with excellent higher mental functions. His mood was somewhat depressed, and he was unkempt and had poor personal hygiene. He explained because of the difficulty of controlling his abdominal pain over the past 2 1/2 years, it had become impossible for him and his wife to remain socially active. For example, to control his pain in social situations with friends, he would often assume awkward or embarrassing postures.
>
> The patient's reliance on Talwin (Pentazocine, a weak narcotic antagonist with some narcotic-like properties) had begun more than 2 years prior to the current treatment. It had been initially prescribed to control pain following abdominal surgery. Mr. X was convinced that this medication was essential for the control of pain and he had spent considerable effort adjusting dosage to his optimal level of 1.25 cc, self-administered intramuscularly, six times daily. Because of the resultant excessive tissue and muscle damage, it had become difficult to find injection sites. The patient insisted that any less than 1.25 cc was almost useless and that more was of no additional value. He had read the early drug literature and was quick to cite evidence that Talwin was not addictive. In addition, Mr. X had no difficulty obtaining his medication by prescription.
>
> Mr. X's primary goal for therapy was to "get more out of life in spite of my pain." He also verbalized the need to control Talwin, but had become highly resistant to any change in his medication regime. (p. 165)

Initially, the treatment program for this patient consisted of self-controlled muscle relaxation. Also, he learned to visualize his pain sensations as "tightening steel bands," which he could "loosen" through relaxation. Although he agreed to change his medication schedule, he was unwilling to have the Talwin dosage of 1.25 cc altered in any manner. Levendusky and Pankratz decided to reduce the dosage of Talwin secretly by gradually substituting a placebo. Within five days, Mr. X unknowingly was receiving pure placebo four times daily. Eventually, the patient was told of the switch, and, although angry, he attributed his improvement to the imagery training and relaxation. At the time of discharge, Mr. X still experienced abdominal pain, but he now had more control over its intensity.

It is poor practice to use deception in the form of placebos to accomplish a therapeutic objective. The Levendusky and Pankratz case study prompted several comments on the use of deception in a treatment setting. The critics all agreed that there were inherent dangers in using deception. For example, if the self-control training had not worked, the patient might have lost faith in the Talwin. Also, the use of placebos can undermine the therapist-patient relationship. That is, even though the deception was for the patient's "own good," he or she will no longer be able to fully trust the therapist, which will harm future efforts at therapeutic intervention. However, the use of deception in this example did illustrate the power of cognitive factors in determining a patient's responsiveness to drug treatment.

Summarizing the current state of the pharmacology of headache is not an easy task. At best, one can say that different drugs seem to be effective for different patients at different times. There is little evidence that the drug industry has achieved its claim of providing highly effective and specialized drugs for patients with different headache symptoms. Ergotamine, the "drug of choice" for patients with migraine symptoms, has been found to be no more effective than a mild analgesic. The traditional diagnostic system has not necessarily improved the practicing physician's ability to treat patients with different headache symptoms. In the end, the physician still must depend heavily on trial and error in combination with knowledge of the patient's response to various medications in the past. Physicians also are caught in the dilemma of having to continually refill and change prescriptions, while knowing that the long-term use of any headache medication is not in their patients' best interests. The phenomenon of ergotamine-induced headache illustrated how the prolonged use of a drug may become part of the very disorder that the drug was designed to prevent. In addition, there are also the problems of drug dependency and side effects that accompany prolonged drug use. At this point, our understanding of drug-behavior interactions is very limited, but it is clear that the current method of controlling headache with medication needs to be changed. All drugs should be administered in a therapeutic context that has as its ultimate goal the prevention of the disorder by the patient himself or herself.

What of Physical Triggers?

The psychobiological model postulates that the conditions controlling headache attacks in the chronic patient operate in a relatively autonomous fashion from both psychological and physical events that exist in the patient's environment. The position presents problems for physicians and patients who believe that physical factors are the main cause or trigger for headache attacks. Medical specialists place a heavy emphasis on the possibility that physical events are responsible for recurrent headache attacks, especially attacks that are associated with migrainous symptoms (Table 5.1). Bright light, weather changes, pollution, and carbon monoxide are often suspected as being responsible for migraine attacks. Foodstuffs are also frequently implicated, with particular attention being directed towards foodstuffs containing monosodium glutamate, alcohol, chocolate, and aged cheese. The menstrual migraine represents another occurrence of headache that is believed to have a physical cause. Women who experience this type of headache see it as being due to hormonal changes that are completely beyond their personal control.

The severity model does not demand that there are *never* physical precipitants of headache attacks. However, it does state that, for most chronic patients, physical triggers are not that significant. This constitutes an important issue because many patients often use the

Table 5.1 Suspected Precipitants of Migraine Attacks

Common Precipitants	Less Common Precipitants
Dietary tyramine, nitrite	Drugs (reserpine, histamine)
Glutamate	Allergic reactions
Oral contraceptives	Humidity
Menstruation	Excessive vitamin A
Hunger	Excessive sleep
Lack of sleep	Environmental chemicals
Bright light, glare	Physical exhaustion
Alcohol	

Adapted from Raskin & Appenzeller, 1980

physical trigger argument as a personal defense against the suggestion that their disorder may have a psychological component. Unfortunately, patients who rigidly adhere to the belief that their attacks constitute an allergy reaction may also find it difficult to conceptualize their disorder in other terms. There are two ways to deal with the issue of physical triggers and headache attacks. First, the data need to be examined critically; second, a framework is needed for understanding what it means when a patient experiences headache attacks in the context of changes in his or her internal/external physical environment. The approach advocated is that physical triggers should not be studied in isolation from the patient's psychobiological makeup. Most patients who have a headache reaction in response to some physical event, such as consuming red wine, do so because they are already headache sufferers and not because of the event per se. Moreover, it will be argued that a headache reaction to weather change, food intake, food abstinence, and menstruation is still a psychobiological reaction and not a parody of an allergic reaction. The shift in emphasis from physical triggers to patient susceptibility again points to the fact that the ultimate control of this disorder lies not in preventing contact between the patient and physical triggers, but in changing his or her susceptibility such that these triggers have little or no impact.

Migraine sufferers often believe that their headaches are triggered by adverse weather conditions, particularly hot dry winds. These hot winds include the Föhn of Switzerland, the Autun of France, the Mediterranean Sirocco, the Chamsin or Sharkiye of the Arab countries, the Argentinian Xonda, the Thar winds of India, the Chinook of Canada, the desert winds of Arizona, and the Santa Ana of Southern California. In one of the few empirical studies of this topic, Wilkinson and Woodrow (1979) monitored weather changes and time of onset of headache attacks in 310 patients who were attending a migraine clinic in London. Each patient was required to record the time of onset of their attacks, and these data were related to several specific weather parameters that included wind direction, wind velocity, barometric pressure, temperature, and humidity. The weather data were provided by a local meteorological office, and readings were obtained for the time of headache onset and for three hours before headache onset to determine if changes in weather conditions before an attack were correlated with the onset of an attack. The researchers found no evidence for the weather hypothesis since none of the weather parameters were systematically related to headache onset. Some of the subjects thought that their headaches predicted bad weather, but no evidence could be found to support this claim. Wilkinson and Woodrow did find that the majority of headache attacks in these chronic headache sufferers occurred in the early hours of the morning, independent of any particular morning. This observation was identical to that made by Bakal, Demjen, and Kaganov (1981) who also found this pattern to be a major characteristic of chronic headache sufferers. However, Wilkinson and Woodrow interpreted their observation differently:

> Some reasons why people develop their headaches between 6:00 and 9:00 A.M. may include a drop in the temperature, a rise in humidity, a change in the CO_2 level during sleep or a rise in the catecholamines... Other possible factors include having to face the trials of the day and coming from the protected atmosphere of a house into the open air. (p. 378)

Although the data are sparse, there is no indication that weather-related factors will ever explain headache attacks in a significant proportion of patients. Much more empirical attention has been directed towards identifying relationships between specific foodstuffs and headache attacks. Four categories of foodstuffs that are frequently mentioned as causing headache are chocolate, cheese and dairy products, citrus fruits, and alcohol (red wine in particular). These substances all contain tyramine and/or phenylethylamine, which are capable of producing vasodilation. Another foodstuff that is hypothesized to precipitate headache through vasodilation is monosodium glutamate (MSG), the suspected trigger of the so-called "Chinese restaurant syndrome." The reason why headache sufferers react to foodstuffs and normals do not is that headache sufferers are presumed to possess a biochemical defect in terms of their body's ability to oxidize tyramine and phenylethylamine.

Chocolate is frequently cited as a trigger of headache, and chocolate is known to contain high amounts of phenylethylamine. Many headache sufferers are convinced that their consumption of chocolate will be followed reliably by a severe headache. In a direct test of this hypothesis, Moffett, Swash, and Scott (1974) identified twenty-five chronic headache sufferers, all of whom initially stated that their headaches could be precipitated by the consumption of chocolate. Subjects were told that they would be required to eat two different kinds of chocolate, but in actuality one of the samples was made from a noncocoa substance that tasted like chocolate. Only a small percentage of the subjects reported experiencing headache following ingestion of the chocolate, and this percentage was not different from that reported for the noncocoa substance. A second study with chocolate (Dalessio, 1980b) involved physicians who suffered from headache and who were convinced that chocolate was a specific trigger of their migraine attacks:

> Four able physicians, experienced in experimental methods, and themselves migraine patients, were the subjects. These four physicians, who were of the opinion that they could predictably produce migraine headache in themselves by eating chocolate in any form and in minimal amounts, were each given a set of lettered, sealed envelopes with the key to the contents held in the laboratory, and unknown to the subject. Each envelope contained either 8 gm powdered chocolate or 8 gm lactose, in eight black capsules. The two sets of capsules were indistinguishable in appearance. Two subjects ingested the contents of an envelope at convenient intervals. One subject ingested the contents of an envelope at regular intervals, three times a week. The fourth subject who commonly awoke on Saturday mornings with a migraine attack after eating chocolate on Friday evening, ingested his capsules on Friday evenings for a period of four months. All were instructed to include no chocolate in their regular diet . . .
>
> It was found in these subjects that headaches sometimes followed the chocolate, sometimes the lactose, but most commonly attacks occurred without reference to the ingestion of capsules. Migraine headaches followed the ingestion of lactose just as frequently as they followed the ingestion of chocolate. The data thus accumulated indicate that in these individuals who considered themselves "allergic" to chocolate even in minimal amounts, the occurrence of their headaches was no more related to the ingestion of chocolate than it was to the ingestion of lactose. (p. 149)

Ziegler and Stewart (1977) administered tyramine and placebo to eighty patients in the context of a double-blind experiment. As mentioned previously, tyramine is a vasodilation-producing substance in a number of foodstuffs that have been suspected of causing headache attacks. The patients were given two capsules, one containing tyramine and the other lactose, and told to take one capsule on a morning that they were in a fasting condition and free of headache and the second capsule on another morning when the same conditions were present. They were asked to report whether or not any headache occurred within twenty-four hours after taking each capsule and, if so, its degree of severity. No headache occurred with either placebo or tyramine in forty-nine patients. Headache occurred after both placebo and tyramine in twelve patients, after placebo but not after tyramine in eleven patients, and after tyramine but not after placebo in eight patients. Seven of the eight patients who responded to tyramine were retested in a second double-blind trial. Five reported no headache, one reported severe headache, and one reported mild headache. There was no evidence that tyramine reliably produced headache attacks; in fact, placebo capsules "produced" more headache attacks than tyramine.

The empirical research has made it clear that headaches do not necessarily occur more frequently in the presence of specific foodstuffs. In addition, there is little indication that headaches that do occur in association with foodstuffs parallel an allergic reaction. An allergic reaction occurs independently of the afflicted person's awareness or nonawareness of the critical substance, and this is not the case with respect to headache attacks. Base rate incidence and superstitious behavior may partially explain why some headache sufferers are convinced of a foodstuff-headache connection. These patients may recall only those attacks that occurred in the presence of a particular food. Also, the critical foodstuff may be consumed in the context of other situational cues that are associated with headache attacks (e.g., wine and cheese parties). Other possible explanations are based on conditioning principles. Jessup (1978) made an analogy between food-related headache attacks and conditioned taste aversion:

> Learned taste aversion occurs when a taste (the conditioned stimulus) is paired with nausea (the unconditioned response) in the classical, Pavlovian conditioning paradigm. Although learned taste aversion violates typical patterns of classical conditioning, the results are congruent with observations by migraineurs concerning suspected food triggers. The interval between the conditioned taste stimulus and the unconditioned response of nausea can be up to 12 hours... Taste aversion is learned in one trial, rather than several, and is exceptionally resistant to extinction. In both humans and animals the learned aversion is specific to the taste that has been followed by nausea, and does not generalize to visual or auditory cues. (p. 229)

An illustration of how resistant this phenomenon is to extinction was provided by Juan Luiv Vives when he wrote, "When I was a boy in Valencia, I was ill of a fever; while my taste was deranged I ate cherries; for many years afterwards, whenever I tasted the fruit, I not only recalled the fever, but also seemed to experience it again."

The link between fasting and headache is also likely psychobiological rather than biochemical in nature. Headaches associated with missing a meal are usually attributed to hypoglycemia (Dexter, Roberts, & Bayer, 1978), and the possibility that such headaches are largely under the control of cognitive variables has never been considered. In a discussion of stress-induced changes of the pituitary-adrenal cortical system, Mason (1975) noted that it is not fasting, but the psychological response to fasting that is critical to initiating hormonal changes. "In fasting, for example, little or no corticosteroid change occurs in monkeys, if fruit-flavored nonnutritive cellulose fiber, i.e., placebo food, is given in place of similarly flavored and shaped regular food pellets, in order to minimize discomfort from emptiness of the gastrointestinal tract and to avoid the psychosocial stimuli associated with sudden deprivation of routine food dispensation by the animal caretaker."

How effective are diets in controlling chronic headache disorders? The evidence is mixed, but it suggests that diets are most effective when patients have strong expectancies that therapeutic changes will occur. Grant (1979) had sixty migraine headache sufferers follow an elimination diet and found that marked reductions in headache activity occurred when these patients avoided foodstuffs containing wheat, orange, eggs, tea, coffee, chocolate, milk, beef, corn, cane sugar, yeast, mushrooms, and peas. Eighty-five percent of the patients were headache free within a few weeks of adopting the diet. It was not possible to determine from Grant's data whether or not these impressive reductions in headache activity were maintained across time. Not only may have the changes been short-term in nature, but they may also have been due to subtle changes in the psychological state of the patients who followed the dietary advice. When psychological influences are ruled out, the effects of diet are far less impressive. For example, Medina and Diamond (1978) minimized specific food-related expectancies by placing migraine patients on three sequential diets, A, B, and C, with each diet being given for six weeks. During diet A, the patients were required to consume foods high in tyramine and phenylethylamine, a diet that should have led to an increase in headache activity. With diet B, the patients were instructed to avoid the foods consumed in diet A; with diet C, the patients were allowed to eat as they pleased. None of the diets had a significant impact on the patients' overall headache activity.

Physical triggers associated with environmental events and/or eating habits are not reliable predictors of headache attacks. Given this to be the case, clinicians might wish to de-emphasize the potential significance these triggers have for understanding headache patients and their symptoms. Too many headache sufferers continue to follow the illusion that some physical substance, in the air, in food, or in their bodies, *must* be responsible for their attacks. Such beliefs recently have been reinforced by a number of articles in popular magazines that are devoted to describing how to control headache by following specific "anti-migraine diets." Helping headache sufferers en masse cannot be accomplished by having the populace continue their search for critical "triggers," for the triggers are not likely to be found. Instead, headache sufferers need to understand how their overall susceptibility to headache (i.e., psychobiological predisposition) renders them susceptible to headache in both the presence and absence of suspected triggers.

Menstrual Migraine

According to Dalton (1973), a link between menstruation and migraine has been suspected since the time of Hippocrates who, it is said, interpreted the menstrual headache as being due to "agitated blood seeking a way of escape." Few female chronic headache sufferers experience their attacks in a fashion that is time-locked to events associated with menses. Moreover, there is no difference in the symptom characteristics of headache sufferers who list menstruation as the principle cause of their attacks and the headache sufferers who list tension as the principal cause of their attacks (Kaganov, 1980). However, there are some women who show a marked increase in headache activity prior to and during menstruation. For example, Dalton found in a selected sample of women that over 60 percent of their attacks occurred during the four days immediately before menstruation and the first four days of menstruation.

Menstrual migraine often is considered part of the *premenstrual syndrome*, a term coined by Frank (1931) to describe a number of negative symptoms that accompany menstruation. The symptoms include depression, irritability, tension, crying, and sometimes headache. Until recently, all of these symptoms were believed to be entirely hormonally based. In fact, this trend continues in headache research as scientists continue to look for biochemical cause-and-effect relationships between headache and menses. The female sex hormones, estradiol and progesterone, are believed to play a major role in initiating the vascular changes of menstrual migraine, although the exact mode of influence is uncertain (Nattero, Bisbocci, & Ceresa, 1979). Researchers dealing with menstruation now recognize that psychological variables are critical determinants of the premenstrual syndrome, and this view also has implications for understanding headache that occurs in phase with menstruation. Ruble and Brooks-Gunn (1979) reviewed existing studies of premenstrual symptoms and concluded that negative affect was not a consistent symptom, since it was sometimes present and sometimes absent. They also noted that mood changes associated with the menstrual cycle were no greater than mood changes associated with other aspects of people's daily lives involving work-related and interpersonal events. In their words, "the data do not seem sufficient to support the commonly held assumptions that psychological fluctuations related to the menstrual cycle do exist for most women, that such fluctuations are tied to underlying hormonal influences, and that they are severe and potentially debilitating."

The most consistently reported symptoms observed by Ruble and Brooks-Gunn were sensory distress and water retention, which are more directly attributable to hormonal influences. If, as argued in the previous chapters, headache is not simply a sensory disorder but includes a large affective and cognitive component, then it seems unreasonable to attribute menstrual headache solely to the same processes that control water retention. Although there are no data available to support this hypothesis, it seems logical that the best way to control menstrual migraine is to alter the patient's overall susceptibility to headache rather than to administer chemicals that alter her hormonal cycle. Many women who experience menstrual headache also experience headache outside their menstrual period.

In summary, it is important that physicians and patients recognize that physical factors are seldom at the basis of chronic headache disorders. Terms like *menstrual migraine, weekend migraine, orgasm migraine, footballer's migraine,* and *hotdog migraine* are misleading because they imply that the identification, control, and avoidance of the relevant triggers are the keys to effective headache management. In discussing the proper workup of a patient, headache experts emphasize the importance of carefully searching with the patient for one or multiple triggers of the attacks. Unfortunately, this style of assessment ignores the basic factors that control the disorder. In dealing with chronic patients, it is important to re-emphasize that no suspected trigger can be specified completely apart from the specification of the psychobiological processes contributing to overall headache susceptibility. Even more important is the fact that chronic headache sufferers do not experience a significant proportion of their headache attacks in the presence of specific physical events or substances. There are no solid theoretical or empirical reasons for continuing to pursue the physical-trigger hypothesis. The hypothesis also lacks credibility with headache sufferers themselves, many of whom have experimented with their physical environments and eating habits without experiencing a significant reduction in headache activity. As will be demonstrated in the next chapters, there are real clinical advantages to abandoning the search for headache triggers in favor of an approach that emphasizes altering a patient's overall susceptibility to headache.

6
Behavioral Approaches to Treatment

The basic premise of the psychobiological model of headache is that chronic headache is the result of two inextricable processes: the individual's failure to cope with less severe headache, accompanied by an increasing involvement and automaticity of the underlying psychological and physiological processes. The model dictates that effective headache control ultimately must come from the headache sufferers themselves, and demands that the behavioral treatment of headache be both encompassing and directed towards teaching patients to recognize and control the various components (cognitive, affective, sensory, physiological) of their disorder. This chapter reviews a number of behavioral techniques that are in use, with the aim of integrating these techniques within the severity model. A specific program of headache management is outlined in the form of a manual in the following chapter.

Biofeedback

The clinical development of biofeedback marked the real beginning of interest in self-control procedures for chronic headache. Initially, biofeedback caused tremendous excitement among therapists because it implied that headache patients could acquire direct voluntary control over the specific physiological systems underlying their headache disorder. In its beginning, biofeedback was used in much

100

the same way drugs are used, the idea being that feedback should focus directly on the physiological system that underlies the disorder. However, more recent research indicates that the exact nature of the feedback modality employed (i.e., EMG feedback, temperature training, EEG feedback) is not critical and that the effects of all forms of biofeedback training may be nonspecific in nature.

The issue of what is learned during biofeedback training is very important for designing effective self-control programs for chronic patients. Both therapist and patient need to have a clear understanding of what can and cannot be expected to happen with this form of self-regulation. There is a growing suspicion that the various types of biofeedback in use for controlling headache all accomplish their therapeutic effects by teaching patients to relax. If this is true, some critics have asked why biofeedback is used at all since relaxation training is an easier and more cost-efficient procedure to use (Beaty & Haynes, 1979). Yates (1980) formulated the mode of action problem in terms of what he called the *specificity/generality assumption*. The specificity assumption was defined as follows:

> If a clinical disorder is correlated with a specific dysfunction in an effector system, then if the dysfunction can be brought under voluntary control and altered to normal levels, there will be a corresponding improvement in the clinical disorder.

Conversely, the generality assumption was defined as follows:

> If a clinical disorder (whether highly specific or more general in nature) exists, successful training in the reduction of levels of activity in any effector system will be accompanied by a corresponding improvement in the clinical disorder.

With respect to headache, specificity refers to the use of EMG feedback for muscle-contraction symptoms and temperature/vasomotor training for migraine symptoms. The early biofeedback studies fostered the impression that headache control was attainable by teaching the patient to directly control his or her physiological functioning. Two publications in particular initiated this belief: the first by Budzynski, Stoyva, and Adler (1970), and the second by Sargent, Green, and Walters (1972). Budzynski et al. used frontal EMG feedback to treat five patients who were suffering from recurrent muscle-contraction headache attacks. During the treatment period, there was a decline in EMG levels and headache activity. The treatment gains were maintained in three patients at the end of three months following treatment. In a similar fashion, Sargent et al. employed hand temperature training to treat a large sample of migraine headache sufferers. The researchers hypothesized that warming the hands resulted in cooling of the forehead and concomitant vasoconstriction of the scalp arteries. The immediate effects of the procedure were impressive since 81 percent of the patients showed improvement. Both groups of investigators had successfully demonstrated that chronic headache sufferers were capable of learning a significant degree of control over their headache disorders. At the same time, however, it was not clear how this control was being achieved, although it was implied that patients were learning to regulate the pathophysiological mechanisms specific to their disorder.

In the intervening period between the publication of these pioneering studies and the present, a very large number of studies have appeared that support the clinical utility of biofeedback training (see reviews by Beaty & Haynes, 1979; Jessup, Neufeld, & Merskey, 1979; Turk, Meichenbaum, & Berman, 1979). However, there are very few researchers today who believe that the effects of biofeedback, although associated with significant reductions in headache activity, are achieved through the direct control of underlying physiological mechanisms. A number of reports in the literature indicate that reductions in headache activity are not necessarily matched by corresponding changes in the physiological mechanisms associated with the biofeedback modality employed.

An example of the lack of specificity found to occur with biofeedback training was provided by Andrasik and Holroyd (1980). In their study, thirty-nine muscle-contraction headache sufferers were assigned to one of four experimental groups. The first group of subjects received conventional EMG feedback training. The next two groups were deceived into thinking that they were lowering frontal EMG, when in fact they were trained either to maintain a stable level or to increase their actual frontal EMG levels. A fourth group was used as a no-treatment control. Analysis of the EMG data indicated that the frontal EMG levels varied in the directions manipulated. However, all three treatment groups showed significant reductions in headache activity, which indicated that learned reductions in EMG activity were not critical to the treatment process. In a discussion of their findings, Andrasik and Holroyd suggested that the improvements were not likely due to expectancy per se. Rather, the biofeedback procedures seemed to have taught these subjects an awareness of some specific strategies for minimizing the frequency of headache attacks. For example, they found that subjects, independent of group membership, devised a number of techniques on their own for controlling headache frequency, such as controlled breathing, refocusing of attention, fantasy, muscle relaxation, and praying. The authors concluded:

> Results from the present study ... indicate that many subjects dealt with their headaches by altering cognitive and behavioral responses to stressful situations ... It may be less crucial that headache sufferers learn to modify EMG activity than it is that they learn to monitor the insidious onset of headache symptoms and engage in some sort of coping response incompatible with the further exacerbation of symptoms. (p. 584)

Although this statement implicates cognitive variables in the mediation of treatment effects associated with biofeedback, it is still important to determine what physiological changes might accompany biofeedback training. Heightened musculoskeletal activity is considered to be a significant component of the predisposition of headache, and the acquisition of effective coping strategies might be expected to be accompanied by reductions in this activity. In their article, Andrasik and Holroyed noted that their headache subjects manifested significantly higher baseline frontal EMG levels when compared to a control group. They did not present data that would allow one to determine whether this frontal EMG activity decreased after the biofeedback training had been completed.

Few studies support the notion that hand warming is associated with cooling of the forehead, or that hand warming per se is the critical variable in temperature feedback training. One study that did support the specificity hypothesis was reported by Turin and Johnson (1976). They found that patients who were trained to lower finger temperature showed no improvement until they were switched to training in raising finger temperature. However, their observation was based on only three patients. Other studies are available that indicate that the direction of temperature training is not critical. Turk et al. cited a study in which one group of migraine patients was trained to raise their finger temperature while a second group was trained to lower their finger temperature. A third group received no training but was required to self-monitor and record headache incidence. All three groups showed similar reductions in headache activity. This study suggests that the effects of hand warming are nonspecific rather than specific in nature.

Additional evidence suggests that the effects of hand warming are not associated with specific changes in the cranial arteries. Sovak, Kunzel, Sternbach, and Dalessio (1978) assessed whether training in hand warming was associated with systematic changes in pulse wave activity recorded from the supraorbital and superficial temporal arteries. Initially, they trained a group of migraine headache sufferers to raise their hand temperature, and ten of twelve patients were eventually able to raise their temperature by at least 2° C. Of the patients who were able to raise their temperature, eight showed a significant reduction in their headache activity. Once the hand warming skill had been acquired, the patients were asked to raise their hand temperature during a session in which simultaneous observations were made of pulse wave activity recorded from the cranial arteries. Hand warming was not accompanied by systematic changes in the pulse wave velocity measures, which indicated that hand warming does not achieve its clinical effects by systematic redistribution of the blood from the head to the hands. However, volitional hand warming was accompanied by a decrease in the patients' heart rate, which led the investigators to propose that volition-induced vasodilation likely occurs in response to a general decrease of tonic sympathetic outflow (i.e., the patients learned to relax).

Other investigators have examined the specificity hypothesis by training patients to directly control vasomotor activity from the cranial arteries. One might expect this to be a more logical choice of feedback modality than the hand, given that migraine is defined as a dysfunction in the regulatory mechanisms that control the responsiveness of cranial arteries. At the same time, keep in mind that this is a presumption only, and it remains to be demonstrated that migraine headache is associated with a vasoconstriction-vasodilation sequence involving the large cranial arteries. It may be that physiological data obtained from the extracranial arteries are as far removed from the physiological mechanisms controlling migraine pain as are data obtained from the hand. In any case, a number of studies have explored the use of cranial feedback for controlling migraine. Friar and Beatty (1976) trained one group of migraine patients to decrease cranial pulse amplitude and another group to decrease finger pulse amplitude. Both strategies were associated with similar reductions in headache frequency, although the group that received cranial feedback experienced fewer "major migraine attacks," which were defined as attacks lasting three hours or more. The authors proposed that training in cranial vasoconstriction allowed the patients to abbreviate rather than prevent their headache attacks. No data were presented that would directly support this hypothesis.

Jessup et al. (1979) reviewed several other studies that have employed cranial biofeedback and, although these studies have demonstrated reductions in headache activity, it is unknown whether or not this form of training represents a more direct form of symptom control than hand warming. One interesting observation that may or may not have a bearing on headache mechanisms is that headache sufferers can apparently learn, through biofeedback, to make differential cranial and peripheral vascular responses. Elmore and Tursky (1981) trained one group of migraineurs to reduce temporal pulse amplitude and another group of migraineurs to increase hand temperature. During the training sessions, temporal pulse amplitude and hand temperature were recorded from all patients. The researchers reported that the greatest changes in the two physiological measures occurred in the modality that was being reinforced. Thus, the greatest decreases in temporal pulse amplitude occurred in the group that was reinforced for decreasing pulse amplitude. The differential effects of training were even more pronounced for the hand temperature data. As illustrated in Figure 6.1, the hand temperature group showed large increases in hand temperature, while the temporal artery group showed decreases in hand temperature. Although the differential training was associated with differential physiological responses, the reductions in headache activity were not substantially different. The temporal artery group reduced their headache frequency from a pretreatment score of 23.3 to 10.3, while the hand warming group reduced their headache frequency from a pretreatment score of 20.0 to 13.0.

Cohen, McArthur, and Rickles (1980) have provided some of the strongest evidence against the notion that biofeedback achieves its effects by teaching patients direct control of underlying physiological mechanisms. After noting that "no matter what modality is chosen—EMG, alpha, temperature, cephalic vasomotor, or combinations of these feedback techniques with other forms of therapy—patients report reductions in the number of headaches experienced," they decided to compare four modalities of feedback in the control of migraine headache attacks. Patients were randomly assigned to one of four biofeedback groups: (1) finger temperature warming, (2) frontal EMG training, (3) EEG (alpha) feedback, and (4) superficial temporal artery feedback. All patients received twenty-four training sessions across an eight- to ten-week period. The authors also corrected a limitation of the majority of biofeedback studies in that they attempted to limit the training procedures exclusively to biofeedback. Unlike other investigators, they did not supplement the training sessions with autogenic training, relaxation exercises, or psychotherapy.

Cohen et al. found no evidence that one form of biofeedback

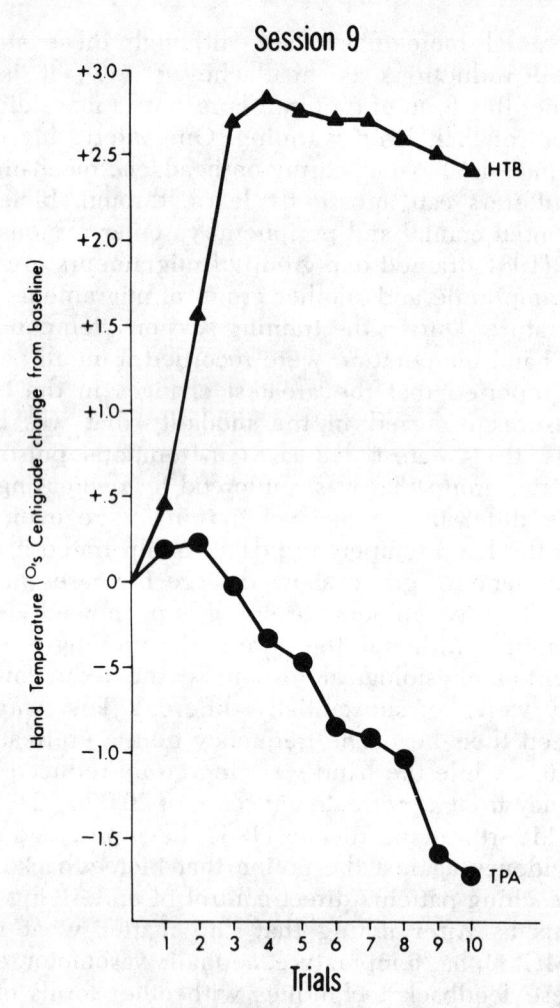

Figure 6.1 Hand temperature changes following hand temperature biofeedback (HTB) and temporal pulse amplitude (TPA) feedback (Elmore & Tursky, 1981). Copyright © 1981 by the American Association for the Study of Headache. Reprinted by permission of the publisher and A. Elmore.

training was better than another. All four groups exhibited similar reductions (approximately 20 percent) in their headache activity following training. The authors also failed to find a correspondence between physiological changes associated with training and changes in headache activity. They proposed that the effects of biofeedback are likely due to the nonspecific effects of relaxation or an increased sense of mastery on the part of the successful patients. It is interesting that the reductions in headache activity were specific to headache frequency and did not occur with characteristics of the actual attacks. That is, following treatment, all patients exhibited fewer attacks, but the attacks that occurred were rated at the same intensity and duration as the attacks that occurred prior to treatment.

In some respects, the specificity/generality issue is a pseudo-issue because headache is not a disorder of a particular effector system. It is a complex psychobiological disorder with both specific and general elements. Moreover, it is still reasonable to assume that systematic changes are occurring at the physiological level, but these changes may not be reflected in the feedback modalities employed. This is particularly true of feedback modalities that are based on the finger and cranial vasculature.

The specificity/generality issue has also been examined in comparisons of biofeedback training with relaxation training. There is no strong evidence that biofeedback is more or less effective than relaxation training in the treatment of either muscle-contraction or migraine headache symptoms (Silver & Blanchard, 1978). In fact, it has been suggested that biofeedback machines are not necessary in the treatment of headache. Biofeedback may not be necessary but it is useful. In discussing the clinical implications of biofeedback, Legewie (1977) made a general comment on how the technology of biofeedback should be viewed, and the comment is most appropriate for understanding the use of biofeedback with headache sufferers:

> In the heyday of biofeedback many of us believed we were on the right path to a new key paradigm for explaining and treating psychosomatic disorders . . . But in spite of the tremendous growth of the biofeedback movement these hopes have proved to be false. Shall we now completely give up the therapeutic application of biofeedback in favor of "better alternatives"? . . . I would like to suggest another approach: We should try to integrate biofeedback as one technique among many others into a more comprehensive treatment approach for psychosomatic disorders . . . Compared with the way biofeedback is commonly used . . . this approach would require a major shift in emphasis. Biofeedback methods would then no longer be the center of focus; rather, they would take on the role of a technical tool which would have to prove itself in competition with other tools. It then becomes essential that on the one hand the biofeedback methods used require less effort than is now the case and on the other hand either the therapist must have thorough training in behavior modification or preferably the biofeedback methods must be used in multidisciplinary treatment centers. (p. 482)

The above statement may seem to have side-stepped rather than solved the problem of how biofeedback achieves its therapeutic effects. This is not true, however, if one views the effects of biofeedback as being indirect rather than direct. With respect to frontal EMG biofeedback, for example, patients do not become aware of the underlying muscle activity per se, nor do they learn to directly regulate this muscle activity. According to Yates (1980), what the patient learns is to re-regulate the servocontrol systems that underlie the activity in the muscles. He uses the concept of servosystem in the same way that physiologists speak of feedback systems as keeping vital body functions within specified limits:

> Consider a subject whose arm hangs loosely and relaxed by his side. The electrical activity of the muscle in such a relaxed state will not be zero but will take an average value resulting from random oscillations about the average value. But this activity is not "uncaused"; it is determined, within the framework adopted here, by the operation of the servocontrol system or systems pertinent to this particular function. This servosystem can be regarded as being constituted of a number of components, each of which may take any one of a range of values; the "resting state" is defined as a particular combination of individual component settings. Suppose now that a decision is reached to increase the tension in that particular muscle. This will be achieved by altering the setting of some (but not necessarily all) of the components of the servosystem, and the particular combination of components which produce particular states of muscle tension is not accessible to "awareness" either. Thus, if the servosystem develops a fault so that an inappropriate combination is set and the muscle malfunctions, there is no reason to suppose that the subject (or patient, as he may now turn out to be) will be able to describe what is wrong (except to say that he gets tension headaches which may be indexed by an increased level of frontalis muscle activity of which the patient is "unaware"). In providing a feedback display of the frontalis muscle activity, the therapist is able to provide the patient with a detailed account of small changes in that activity. But what the patient learns when he produces changes in the muscle activity which are reflected in the feedback display is not a greater "awareness" of his muscle activity. *What he learns is the "language" of the servocontrol system; that is, how to modify the relative settings of the components of the control system so as to produce the appropriate muscle activity in a specified situation.* The feedback display is merely a device to teach the patient about his control systems. (p. 463)

This position has implications for understanding the approach to be used in the treatment of chronic headache patients. First, there is no *a priori* reason why biofeedback training should be more or less effective than relaxation training. For example, a patient with sustained muscle tightness in the shoulder/neck region might be expected to benefit equally from either procedure, *if* the patient is taught the importance of developing personal strategies for continually regulating these sensations. Second, the emphasis on higher-order servocontrol mechanisms points to the necessity of teaching patients to gain control of more than peripheral physiological response mechanisms. Headache patients also must learn to regulate the cognitive component of their disorder. In fact, there is a strong possibility that the effectiveness of biofeedback is largely determined by its ability to make patients aware of the importance of altering the thoughts and feelings that precede and accompany their headache attacks. A recent study by Sovak, Kunzel, Sternbach, and Dalessio (1981) is supportive of such an hypothesis. In this study, twenty-nine female migraine headache sufferers were given training in hand warming, while another twenty patients were given a standard form of drug treatment. MMPI data were collected on all patients, both before and after treatment. Although all the biofeedback-treated patients demonstrated the ability to raise their hand temperature, only half the patients showed significant reductions in their headache activity. The patients who improved also showed significant reductions in their scores to the hypochondriasis, hysteria, and depression scales of the MMPI. The unimproved patients showed no change in their MMPI scores. Apparently, the successful patients were able to evolve a number of coping strategies over and above the strategies learned in the biofeedback training sessions, while the unsuccessful patients were not. The fact that only half of the patients made this transition indicates the limitation of attempting to achieve this goal with biofeedback training alone.

Cognitive Skills Training

The view that biofeedback represents a rather narrow and mechanical approach to headache therapy was first made by Miechenbaum (1976). He noted that the biofeedback approach fails to appreciate that headache is determined by a complex set of responses, including cognitive, affective, and sensory, as well as physiological components. Meichenbaum proposed that a more successful approach to self-management might be achieved by designing programs that viewed therapy as a three-stage process. First, the patient must become aware of his or her maladaptive intrapersonal and interpersonal behaviors. That is, the patient must observe the role that thoughts, feelings, behaviors, physiological responses, and reactions of others play in maintaining his or her disorder. This process is facilitated by means of a conceptualization process of how the patient views his or her problem. The process of self-observation acts as a stimulus for the patient to engage in incompatible thoughts and behaviors, which constitutes the second stage of the treatment process. Finally, the patient must transfer these cognitive skills to his or her natural environment. What the patient says to himself or herself (e.g., his or her appraisal, attributions, self-evaluations) about his or her behavior will influence the amount of transfer of treatment that occurs.

Several publications now have appeared that support the clinical utility of treating headache sufferers within a cognitive behavioral framework. Mitchell and White (1977) developed an elaborate skills training program that they successfully applied to a small number of migraine patients. The program mirrored very closely the treatment sequence Meichenbaum outlined. As stated by the authors, the goal of the program was to help migraine patients "analyze and identify problems in their own personal environments and behaviors (both overt and covert), to work out their own management strategies, and to self-apply control techniques aimed at modifying both their environment and their reactions to that environment." During the first stage of the program, patients were simply required to monitor their headache activity. They were also told that migraine headaches were due to certain predisposing factors, namely genetic and constitutional, and that there was nothing they could do to control the onset of migraine once the biochemical process had started. However, they could learn to monitor and prevent the occurrence of stressful events that triggered the biochemical process. Following the self-observation and conceptualization phase, patients were given training in cue-controlled progressive muscle relaxation, mental relaxation, and self-desensitization. These skills were designed to be used in the context of situational stress. A second skill-acquisition stage was used with only three patients and consisted of training in thirteen additional self-control techniques (e.g., rational thinking, assertion training, imaginal modeling).

Mean headache frequency remained unchanged among all patients during the self-observation period, which indicated that self-monitoring alone was not sufficient to reduce migraine headache attacks. However, the two skill-acquisition phases resulted in significant decreases in headache frequency. Patients who received only the first stage of training showed a decrease of at least 50 percent in the frequency of their attacks over a sixty-week period. Patients who received the entire program showed a 75 percent reduction in their headache frequency across the same period. The results of their study are even more impressive when it is recognized that virtually the entire program was conducted by audio taped instructions.

Holroyd, Andrasik, and Westbrook (1977) also developed a cognitive skills training program for muscle-contraction headache sufferers. Their program emphasized directly the role that cognitions play in stress reactions and subsequent headache attacks:

> The rationale for treatment emphasized that disturbing emotional and behavioral responses are a direct function of specifiable maladaptive cognitions. It was emphasized that tension headache results from psychological stress and that stress responses are determined by cognitions about an event or situation. Several concrete examples were provided to illustrate the variety of events that can be perceived as stressful by different individuals and the way in which cognitions can induce psychological stress and headache. Unreasonable expectations (that one should be perfect or liked by everyone) were discussed and the manner in which they predispose individuals to experience stress was illustrated. Thus clients were encouraged to attribute the cause of their headaches to relatively specific cognitive aberrations rather than to external stimuli or complex inner dispositions. (p. 125)

Holroyd et al. compared the effectiveness of their cognitive procedure with EMG biofeedback training. The group receiving cognitive skills training was initially trained to identify: (1) cues that trigger tension and anxiety; (2) the way they responded when anxious; (3) their thoughts prior to, during, and following their becoming tense; and (4) the way these cognitions appeared to contribute to their headache attacks. The results indicated that cognitive skills training was more effective in reducing headache activity than biofeedback training, both at post-treatment and at fifteen-month follow-up.

In a second study, Holroyd and Andrasik (1978) made a comparison between specific cognitive skills training and headache discussion. One group of headache sufferers was given training in the same cognitive procedures that were used in their initial study. A second group of patients received training in what was termed *headache discussion*. The treatment consisted of a discussion of the historical roots of their symptoms ("Your anxiety appears to be a natural reaction to the way you were treated as a child"). The rationale presented for this treatment also described headaches as resulting from psychological stress, but it emphasized that feelings of distress would improve if patients understood the underlying source of their problems. Apparently, the latter patients when left more to their own resources were able to evolve strategies that were as effective as those used by patients who received more specific training, since both groups showed similar degrees of improvement following treatment. The authors noted that patients in the headache discussion group devised coping strategies that were quite similar to the strategies taught to the cognitive control group. In some instances, however, the patients left to their own devices developed coping techniques that were quite unique. One patient began praying when she noted cognitive symptoms of distress, while another patient imaginally engaged in karate exercises. These observations led the investigators to conclude that "It may be less crucial to provide clients with specific coping responses than to insure that they monitor the insidious onset of symptoms and are capable of engaging in some sort of cognitive or behavioral response incompatible with the further exacerbation of symptoms."

As indicated previously, chronic headache patients experience the majority of their attacks in the absence of external precipitants; consequently, they may have difficulty relating to management procedures that emphasize the importance of identifying situational stressors. Bakal, Demjen, and Kaganov (1981) developed a cognitive intervention program that places a heavy emphasis on modifying sensory and distress reactions associated with headache susceptibility and headache attacks. The patients used in the study were all in a chronic condition, and many had tried, without success, to control their attacks with self-hypnosis, biofeedback, acupuncture, and dieting.

The treatment procedure consisted of three overlapping phases. (A complete description of the program is presented in the next chapter.) The first phase began with having each patient monitor his or her headache activity on the self-observation headache frequency record. Each patient monitored his or her headache activity on a daily basis for a three-week period. In addition to providing baseline data, the self-observation period was used to have patients begin observing the sensations, thoughts, and feelings that precede and accompany their headache attacks. The self-observation period also marked the beginning of having the patients learn the necessity of becoming active collaborators in the treatment process.

The self-observation period was followed by eleven treatment sessions that were conducted individually with each patient on a weekly basis. Throughout all sessions, patients were encouraged to acquire a new understanding of their headache condition, an understanding that permitted them to view previously undifferentiated attacks as consisting of a number of smaller and describable components. During the initial session, the therapist discussed physiological mechanisms that may underlie headache susceptibility (e.g., heightened muscle activity in neck and head regions) and how this susceptibility may be exacerbated by sensations and cognitions that precede and accompany headache attacks. Relaxation training was also introduced during the first session and continued during the second session, after which a relaxation tape was provided for home practice. Following relaxation training, each patient received five sessions of EMG biofeedback training. Both forms of training were used in the context of behavioral assessment rather than in the context of direct muscle control. That is, patients were encouraged to observe changes in bodily sensations, thoughts, and feelings that accompanied any changes in their EMG levels.

The second phase, called the skill-acquisition phase, consisted of teaching specific coping skills that enabled the patients to deal with the previously identified components of their headache attacks. During sessions eight through eleven, patients were given training in the use of attention focusing, imagery production, and thought management (Turk, 1978). Transfer of the acquired skills from the clinical setting to the patient's natural environment constituted the last phase of the program. Graduated home assignments were given in order to consolidate the newly acquired skills and to facilitate generalization of these skills to the natural environment. Post-treatment and follow-up data were collected by having the patients monitor their headache activity for fourteen days immediately following the last session and for an additional fourteen days six months after treatment had terminated.

Overall, the treatment procedure was found to be highly effective, both immediately at the end of treatment and at the six-month follow-up. For the entire sample, the number of daily headache hours was reduced by 57.1 percent. A subsample of the group that had completed six-month follow-up had maintained its improvement. Although the procedure was highly effective overall, there were large differences in the degree to which individual patients benefited from the procedure. Some patients showed no improvement while other patients showed a complete disappearance of their problem. Headache diagnosis was not found to be predictive of patient responsiveness to the program, a finding that was encouraging for the severity model. Similarly, head pain locations and symptoms reported on the self-observation record did not predict treatment responsiveness, nor did sex, age, and years of reported problem headache. However, an incidental observation revealed a patient variable that proved to be highly predictive of treatment effectiveness/ineffectiveness. It was noticed that patients with continuous or near-continuous pain during the waking hours showed little change in headache activity from pretreatment to post-treatment. To empirically demonstrate this observation, the patients were grouped on the basis of their daily pretreatment headache scores into three groups: (1) those who experienced less than 8.0 average hours of head pain per day; (2) those who experienced between 8.0 to 14.9 hours of head pain per day; (3) those who experienced 15.0 or greater hours of head pain per day. The first two groups, representing what may be called episodic headache disorders, showed reduction of 52 percent and 61 percent, respectively, in their post-treatment headache hours. The third group, representing continuous pain, showed a reduction of only 11 percent in post-treatment headache activity. The cognitive behavioral intervention procedure was clearly not effective for chronic headache patients with continuous or near-continuous pain during the waking hours.

The results of the Bakal et al. study provided strong support for the use of cognitive behavior therapy in the treatment of chronic headache. The results were especially encouraging since the patients used in the study had suffered from headaches of longstanding duration that had become difficult to control with medication. The cognitive treatment program had two main objectives: (1) to provide patients with a psychobiological understanding of their disorder, and (2) to provide patients with a number of cognitive strategies for regulating the frequency and severity of headache attacks. It was hypothesized that treatment effectiveness was largely determined by the extent to which the behavioral procedures encouraged patients to develop personal strategies for regulating the psychobiological processes controlling their headache attacks. Herein lies the major advantage of the cognitive behavioral perspective, as it explicitly encourages patients to generate their own individually tailored coping packages. To illustrate, a female migraine patient found that practicing relaxation training caused her to have more frequent rather than less frequent headache attacks. However, she did benefit from training in attention-diversion by developing a personal strategy of "becoming busy" whenever she sensed that a headache attack was imminent. Her headache attacks were regularly preceded by scintillating scotoma that she eventually used as cue to begin practicing her attention-diversion skills. At six-month follow-up, she had not reported a single headache attack, although her scintillating scotoma continued to occur as frequently and as regularly as before treatment. A two-year follow-up revealed that her control of the headache attacks had been maintained and also that the visual symptom was beginning to occur less frequently and less distinctly.

No adequate explanation was available to explain the failure of the procedure to assist headache patients with continuous or near-continuous pain. Self-control procedures are more effective when a disorder is episodic rather than continuous in nature. With continuous pain headache sufferers, it is unknown whether the physiological mechanisms contributing to their disorder are associated with structural changes or whether such patients simply have difficulty accepting the behavioral model being offered.

Hypnosis as a Form of Cognitive Control

Family practitioners often use or recommend hypnosis as a procedure to help their patients manage with chronic headache. The use of hypnosis in general medical practice was sanctioned by the American Medical Association in 1958 and by the British Medical Association in 1955. The early literature emphasized the use of hypnosis to help headache sufferers acquire insight into emotional conflicts that were presumed to be at the basis of their pain disorder (Blumenthal, 1963). However, the psychoanalytic position has given way to a view that is quite compatible with the cognitive approach to headache management. In most circles, hypnosis is now seen as constituting a cognitive tool for teaching patients to minimize the pain during attacks and to become more aware of psychological events that lead to attacks. Thus, much of what happens during the administration of hypnosis takes place outside of the induction procedure itself.

In treating chronic headache sufferers, some specialists have used the suggestion of direct physiological control. For example, Harding (1961) gave his migraine patients the hypnotic suggestion that they could abort the pain of a migraine attack by visualizing the blood vessels in their head growing smaller and returning to normal. Anderson, Basker, and Dalton (1975) used the following similar suggestion:

> Migraine is caused by ... and always made worse by tension ... thus making the arteries in the head congested and large. I want you to visualize the arteries in the head ... picture them large and throb-

bing ... now, as you relax and become less tense ... each day ... your arteries become smaller and smaller ... more normal. The arteries stay normal ... and your head feels comfortable. (p. 51)

Both Harding and Anderson et al. reported the hypnotic procedure to be effective. For example, Anderson et al. reported that ten of twenty-three patients were completely free of migraine attacks during the last three months of their one-year clinical trial. Several other studies that have found positive effects with hypnosis training have recently been reviewed by De Piano and Salzberg (1979).

Is hypnosis a unique form of cognitive control? This question still has not been settled satisfactorily although, as suggested before, most specialists believe that it is not. Andreychuk and Skriver (1975) compared self-hypnosis with hand warming and alpha biofeedback training in the management of headache symptoms. The hypnotic procedure was described as involving "relaxation instruction, visual imagery, verbal reinforcers, and direct suggestions for dealing with pain." Interestingly, the three techniques produced similar reductions in post-treatment headache activity. Of additional interest was the observation that highly suggestible patients responded better than less suggestible patients, regardless of the type of treatment received. The highly suggestible patients showed an improvement of 71 percent and the less suggestible patients showed an improvement of 41.4 percent. Barber, Spanos, & Chaves (1974) maintain that hypnosis is no more effective in the production of relaxation than mere instruction to sit quietly, as indicated by physiological criteria. And yet, those familiar with the procedure have developed a variety of strategies that may be effective only when implemented through hypnosis. Ansel (1977) reported a case study involving a migraine patient who was having difficulty implementing the hypnotic suggestion to warm her hand. He described his solution to the problem as follows:

While working with her, I recalled witnessing, as a youngster, a trick performed by another youth in which he rapped the base of several fingers with a comb, producing no apparent effect. However, he then proceeded to fling his arm around in a rapid, circular motion, causing a pronounced influx of blood into the hand. This resulted in the appearance of minute trickles of blood where the teeth of the comb had almost imperceptibly weakened the skin at the base of the fingers— much to the astonishment of several youthful onlookers.

I asked [the patient] to now duplicate this motion, first with one arm and then with the other, omitting, of course, the use of the comb. There was an immediate and striking response. The dominant right hand, used first, became quickly engorged, grew noticeably warmer, and was quite red in color, especially in comparison with the icy coldness and pallor of the left hand. . . . Duplication of this motion quickly brought about similar changes in the left hand. [The patient] was encouraged to concentrate on the sensation of blood surging into the hand. (p. 69)

According to Ansel, the patient was able to use this sensory experience in a fashion that facilitated production of the hand warming response to subsequent suggestions in hypnosis. This case study suggests that the real value of hypnosis may lie not in the induction procedures but in the imagination and creativity of the hypnotists who devise these strategies.

Spanos and his colleagues (Spanos, Radtke-Bodorik, Ferguson, & Jones, 1979) have added another dimension to hypnosis research, a dimension that is extremely relevant to the present thesis. Spanos has stated that the effectiveness or ineffectiveness of hypnosis and suggestion procedures in the control of pain are largely determined by the patient's ability or inability to generate pain-control cognitions. Since these cognitions are not necessarily provided by the hypnotist, it is often left to the patient to evolve his or her own strategies for minimizing the pain. The argument is important because it reinforces the notion that hypnotic pain control is not a passive automatic process but requires active cognitive effort on the part of the hypnotized patient. To demonstrate this phenomenon, they conducted an experiment with the coldpressor test in which they had subjects place their hand in ice water with the suggestion that the hand would gradually become numb and insensitive until no pain was experienced. No suggestions were given as to how this analgesic state was to be achieved. Following the experiment, the subjects were interviewed in order to determine how they succeeded or failed at this task. The successful subjects were found to have reduced the pain experience by generating a variety of cognitive strategies of their own invention. Some subjects used distraction ("I was counting in my head, sort of counting off seconds"), others used pain-incompatible imagery ("I imagined that the arm was dead"), and still others used imagery associated with relaxation ("I was imagining lying on the beach basking in the sun"). Unsuccessful subjects (labelled by the authors as "catastrophizers") generated thoughts and feelings as well but with a different emphasis. They used cognitions that focused on and exaggerated the unpleasantness of the situation ("I kept thinking I can't stand this much longer, I want to get out").

It is significant that the main dependent variables in studies dealing with hypnosis and headache have not involved changes in the pain experienced during attacks but rather changes in the overall susceptibility to headache attacks. The successful application of hypnosis lies not so much with its ability to abort attacks that have begun but to reduce the number of attacks that occur. The psychobiological processes underlying headache susceptibility are somehow normalized in those patients who find the technique useful. The nature of this normalization process needs investigation because it may be more important than the hypnotic procedure itself. Some headache sufferers are capable of making therapeutic changes to their system without direction, but many others are not. As with biofeedback, headache sufferers who cannot make the transition from the technique to daily functioning will not likely benefit from training in hypnosis. Hypnosis should be used only as a tool to help patients recognize and alter the complex processes that control their disorder. Whether hypnosis is more effective than other self-control techniques or whether it is more suitable for some patients than others are issues that require empirical examination. Many hypnosis researchers believe that good candidates for hypnosis are patients who are highly suggestible, but such patients may be equally good candidates for cognitive behavioral intervention. Also, too much emphasis has been placed on the presence/absence of the trait of "suggestibility," since not all highly hypnotizable individuals are successful in reducing their pain, nor are all less hypnotizables unsuccessful (Hilgard, 1975). A more positive approach would be to explore the use of hypnosis in conjunction with cognitive behavioral strategies, especially with patients with whom the latter strategies have proved ineffective. For example, hypnosis might represent a powerful tool for breaking the continuous pain cycle that characterizes some headache sufferers. If successful, the application of hypnosis would then make it much easier to teach these patients additional coping strategies to prevent the further recurrence of chronic headache.

Summary

In the 1940s, Harold Wolff insightfully commented that the effective management of chronic headache requires that the patient recognize at the outset that "there is no easy road to the goal he wishes to achieve, and especially must he appreciate that anything out of a bottle can offer him no more than transient help." Exactly the same conclusion can be reached with the use of behavioral techniques such as relaxation training, biofeedback, and hypnosis. Just as there is no magical chemical cure for headache, there is also no magical behavioral cure for headache. This means that unless chronic headache sufferers learn to identify and regulate the sensations, thoughts, and feelings that have become intertwined with the physiochemical mechanisms that control their headache syndrome, the benefits of self-control techniques can be expected to be transitory.

The behavioral treatment of headache not only must be encompassing, but also must focus on altering the psychobiological processes that maintain the disorder. The approach does not demand that headache sufferers require a major overhaul of their personalities and life situations. Not only is psychotherapy, in the traditional sense, unnecessary, but there is no evidence that it is capable of teaching patients to live "happily ever after." Most people in our society continually find themselves confronted with life problems with which they must cope and headache represents just one more problem. The cognitive approach to headache management has led to the exciting possibility that the psychobiological processes controlling chronic headache can be identified and reversed. However, enthusiasm for the approach must be tempered with an awareness that long-term follow-up data with the procedure are still not available. Such data are critical because it is suspected that the permanent control of headache requires that patients learn their newly acquired skills to such an extent that the self-regulatory processes become an automatic aspect of their daily functioning.

7
A Manual for the Cognitive Behavioral Treatment of Chronic Headache

This chapter outlines a cognitive behavioral treatment program for chronic headache sufferers. The program was developed over the course of several years and has been successfully administered to a large number of headache patients with varying symptomatologies and with various diagnoses. The program is based on techniques that are in common use in behavioral medicine and is relatively easy to implement in clinical and hospital settings. The guiding premise behind the program is that self-regulation of headache depends on the patient's ability to recognize and control the thoughts, feelings, sensations, and physiological processes that contribute both to headache susceptibility and to headache attacks. Because chronic headache is often characterized by attacks that occur in the absence of precipitating stress, the primary emphasis of the program is on teaching patients to recognize and regulate the psychobiological processes that maintain their disorder. Situational and antecedent stressors are de-emphasized in favor of headache-related distress that is viewed as a major component of the chronic headache syndrome.

In broad terms, the program has two main objectives: (1) to provide headache sufferers with a psychobiological understanding of their disorder, and (2) to provide headache sufferers with the means of developing their own strategies for regulating the frequency and severity of headache attacks. The program consists of twelve individual treatment sessions, conducted at weekly intervals.

Each session is designed to last forty to fifty minutes. Although the program is time-consuming and demanding, it is remarkably effective in producing clinical gains, which is sufficient reward for the effort required.

The program is described such that it should be relatively easy to implement in other behavioral medicine centers. Patient successes as well as patient failures are discussed in the hope that this information will minimize the beginning frustrations that inevitably occur with the implementation of new programs. It is hoped that the program will serve primarily as a model of treatment and encourage experimentation with additional techniques. No claims are made for the necessity of adhering rigidly to the treatment format. Some patients exhibit clinical improvement after a few treatment sessions, although most patients require the entire therapy program.

The program adheres very closely to the cognitive self-control theory of Meichenbaum (1976). Meichenbaum proposed that behavioral treatment be viewed as a three-stage process involving an observational phase, an educational phase, and a skill-acquisition phase. During the observational phase, the patient and the therapist collect data that are relevant to the presenting problem. During the educational phase, a common conceptual framework is developed for understanding the problem. Finally, during the skill-acquisition phase, the patient learns to modify the cognitions and behaviors associated with his or her problem. The application of this theory to the control of chronic pain disorders was facilitated by Genest (1977) and Turk (1978, 1980). The experimental and theoretical work of these investigators provided the rationale and clinical tools that are used in the present program.

The treatment program uses several specific cognitive and behavioral techniques, but the techniques primarily illustrate the parameters that need to be controlled and the kinds of strategies that may be employed to achieve the control. Although psychobiological processes are assumed to be similar across headache patients, each patient is also assumed to be a unique individual. Patients vary not only in terms of their presenting symptomatology, but also in terms of their thoughts, feelings, and preferred ways of coping. The entire program adheres to the principle that therapy must be individually tailored for each patient. Adhering to this principle necessitates that the therapist and patient evolve a shared conceptualization of the headache disorder. Cameron (1978) stressed the significance of this approach to therapy as follows:

> ... the client is likely to be resistant to attempts to educate him if he believes that the therapist is mechanically imposing a prefabricated conceptualization upon his problem, in a "hard sell" fashion. One of the major hazards of using a "hard sell" approach is that the client may easily come to believe that he is unable to challenge the therapist's conceptualization. The therapist appears to him to be so invested in his point of view that any questioning of the conceptualization would be futile. As a consequence, the client may be overtly compliant, but harbor serious reservations or misunderstandings that are never dealt with. In order to please the hard-sell therapist, the client may engage in much head-nodding even though he doesn't comprehend, may turn in bogus homework assignments, and even report counterfeit improvement. While it is undoubtedly advantageous for a therapist to be enthusiastic with clients, clients need to believe that they can honestly report lack of understanding, misgivings, or lack of progress. (p. 243)

An example of how a didactic approach to therapy may fail comes from a patient who had received fifty-two sessions of hand warming training at another clinic. She had no idea of what hand warming had to do with counteracting her headache attacks. Furthermore, she could not learn, even after a year's practice, to raise her hand temperature. The therapist allegedly told the patient that she was not able to "turn on the appropriate division of her nervous system" and that nothing further could be done. The patient was afraid to challenge the therapist's position and felt quite hopeless and confused with her failure to do whatever it was that the therapist believed was necessary. It is extremely important that the therapist and patient have a common understanding of the treatment process and that they work together in designing a program with which the patient is comfortable.

The requirement that the therapist and patient evolve, during the course of therapy, a shared conceptualization of the headache disorder makes the writing of a step-by-step manual difficult. Although the therapist may comprehend the changes required by the psychobiological model, each patient will have to achieve this understanding on his or her own terms. This can only be accomplished if the therapist is skillful in identifying the resources that the patient brings to therapy as well as the resources in which the patient is deficient. Patient strengths and weaknesses cannot be specified in advance and must be identified as part of the treatment procedure. In the same fashion, progress or lack of progress associated with specific sessions will have a bearing on what is done in succeeding sessions, and for this reason there are no firm boundaries between the sessions. The manual is presented only as a guide for helping therapists and patients discover the means to recognize and regulate the complex psychobiological processes that control the headache disorder. A schematic of the overall program is presented in Figure 7.1.

The Patient's Conceptualization of Headache

No patient is accepted into the program until he or she has received a neurological examination. It is also recommended that the patient remain in the care of his or her physician and that the physician be provided with an explanation of the rationale and the goals behind the program. The purpose of the opening treatment session is to acquire some understanding of how the patient conceptualizes his or her disorder and to provide the patient with a brief understanding of the objectives behind the program. The session begins with a discussion of the headache itself, with the therapist directing questions towards determining when headache first became a problem and if

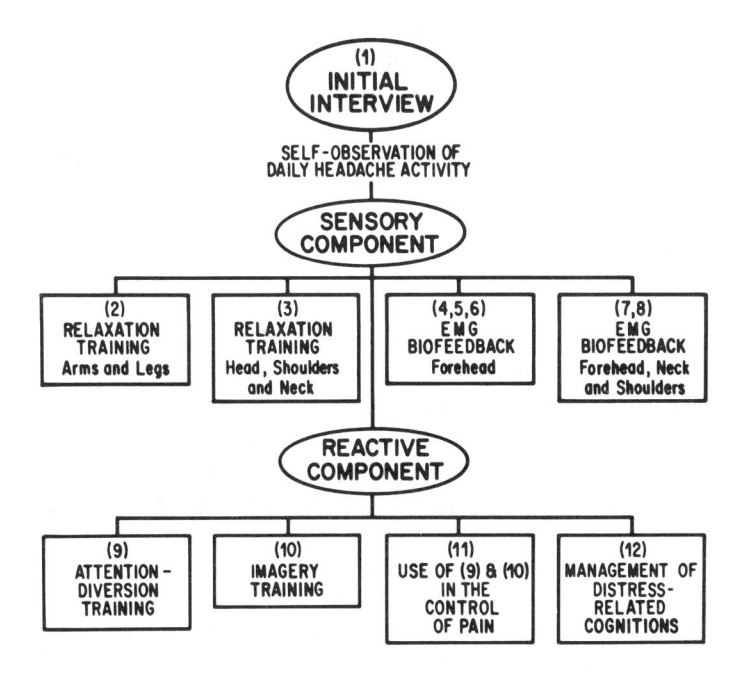

Figure 7.1 Outline of cognitive behavioral treatment program.

any specific circumstances were associated with its onset and change in severity over the years. The therapist is not probing for a cause but is simply trying to formulate some understanding of how the patient views the disorder.

Severe headaches generally follow a progressive course of development, beginning in childhood in the form of occasional headache and then increasing in frequency and severity over the years. Thus, few chronic headache sufferers believe that one event or multiple events occasioned the onset of their disorder. There are instances where the transition from nonproblem to problem headache is sudden and occurs concomitantly with some event, such as marriage, divorce, or increased work responsibilities. Only a small number of headache patients have strong views concerning "triggers" for their attacks. Most patients simply feel that something is wrong without knowing what it may be.

The next portion of the interview deals directly with characteristics of the patient's headache attacks. The patient is asked to describe the attacks in terms of frequency, time of onset, and degree of variation from one attack to the next. Also explored are the quality of pain experienced (dull/aching or throbbing), locations of pain involved, and whether the pain is intermittent or continuous. Additional questions deal with the nature of symptoms that occur prior to the onset of pain and during the actual headache attack. It is important to query if persistent sensations of tightness and pressure are present, especially during periods outside of the headache attack. Unless prompted, patients will often fail to mention the presence of these symptoms.

An inquiry of the methods of controlling headaches that the patient has used in the past and is using in the present is made next. Drug usage is determined, but no recommendations are given for change. The patient is told that, if the program is successful, he or she will eventually require less medication. Generally, patients are eager to find alternatives to using drugs. The patient is also asked to describe any self-control procedures that he or she has used in the past either to reduce the severity of an attack or to eliminate the attack completely. If self-control procedures (e.g., hypnosis, relaxation exercises) have been used in the past, the therapist explores how the procedures were used and why, in the patient's view, the procedures failed. Some patients report using self-control procedures of their own creation, such as directing attention to other matters or finding a quiet place to rest. However, they seldom have considered using such strategies in a systematic fashion. Identifying self-control strategies in use by the patient is important because the same strategies can be incorporated within the treatment program at a later stage.

Following the discussion of the patient's history and current situation, the therapist provides an explanation of the rationale behind the present program. Rather than emphasize situational antecedents of headache attacks, the patient is simply told that the disorder has acquired a life of its own and is now operating independently from events that trigger headache attacks in less severe headache sufferers. Some patients will report situations that reliably exacerbate their headache condition, and in such cases the therapist determines the impact of the headache on the patient's behavior in the situation. For example, if a headache develops in response to a specific work or home situation, it is important to determine the particular aspects of the situation that contribute to the attack and how the accompanying pain and misery interferes with the patient's ability to function in the situation. The patient is told that headache attacks that occur in the presence or absence of specific events may be viewed as consisting of two components, a sensory component and a reactive component. The sensory component consists of the sensation of pain that is largely determined by changes in the underlying muscles and vessels of the head. The reactive, or cognitive, component consists of the thoughts and feelings that accompany headache attacks. The therapist indicates that during the initial sessions therapy will be directed towards altering the sensory component through relaxation and biofeedback training, and during later sessions additional strategies will be provided for dealing with the reactive component.

The session ends with the first assignment, which is to have the patient monitor his or her daily headache activity for a three-week period. He is provided with a sample headache frequency record, as shown in Figure 7.2, and a typed explanation of how to complete the record. The explanation is rehearsed as follows:

> You are to monitor for the next three weeks your daily headache activity. By doing so you will come to understand your headaches better and provide us with important information which we will discuss together during the treatment sessions. Here is an example of a completed headache frequency record. On these cards you are to record the intensity, location, and time of onset of your headache attacks, as well as the symptoms which you experience. You can also keep a record of the amount and kind of medication which you consume during the day. You may also wish, in the Notes section, to write down any thoughts or feelings which you may have during an attack. The inten-

sity of pain is to be rated from 0 to 5 where 0 refers to no pain; 1 to mild pain (only aware of it when attention is directed towards it); 2 to discomforting pain (can be ignored); 3 to painful pain (hurts but does not interfere with activities); 4 to severe pain (difficult to concentrate on tasks); and 5 to intense, incapacitating pain. To illustrate the procedure, let us work through this example. Between 8:00 A.M. and 10:00 A.M. the individual began to experience neck pain on both sides (1,11) at a mild intensity (1). Between 10:00 A.M. and 12:00 A.M., the head pain had extended to the eyes (6,16) and was experienced as discomforting (2). From 12:00 A.M. to 2:00 P.M. the pain at both locations increased in intensity such that it was now severe (4). At this time, two Fiorinal tablets were taken. From 2:00 P.M. to 4:00 P.M. the headache decreased in intensity. During the day the individual also experienced sensations of tightness and pressure, throbbing pain, light sensitivity and nausea. Please make certain to record the symptoms which are experienced during the headache attacks. Feel free to use the Notes section, as in the example, to provide information concerning what you are doing and feeling during the day.

It is recommended that the self-observation procedure be employed with each patient. It provides an efficient means of quantifying treatment effectiveness, and serves as a valuable clinical assessment tool. By monitoring headache activity, many patients come to appreciate for the first time that their headache activity can be analyzed into components, which serves to reinforce the notion that self-control is possible. The requirement of self-observation serves as a signal to the patients that they must become active collaborators in the treatment process. Finally, the self-observation records can be used as a point of discussion throughout the treatment program.

Relaxation/Biofeedback Training

The first skills-training session begins with a review of the self-observation headache records. The patient now has considerable skill in analyzing his or her attacks in terms of locations and symptoms involved, time of onset, duration of attacks, variation in attacks, etc. The therapist discusses the headache patterns reported on the cards and ensures that the patterns observed are representative of the patient's problem. At this point, some patients remain suspicious that the purpose of therapy is to probe for psychological reasons for the affliction, which in their view represents a contradiction with their personal experience with headache. The fact that the self-observation

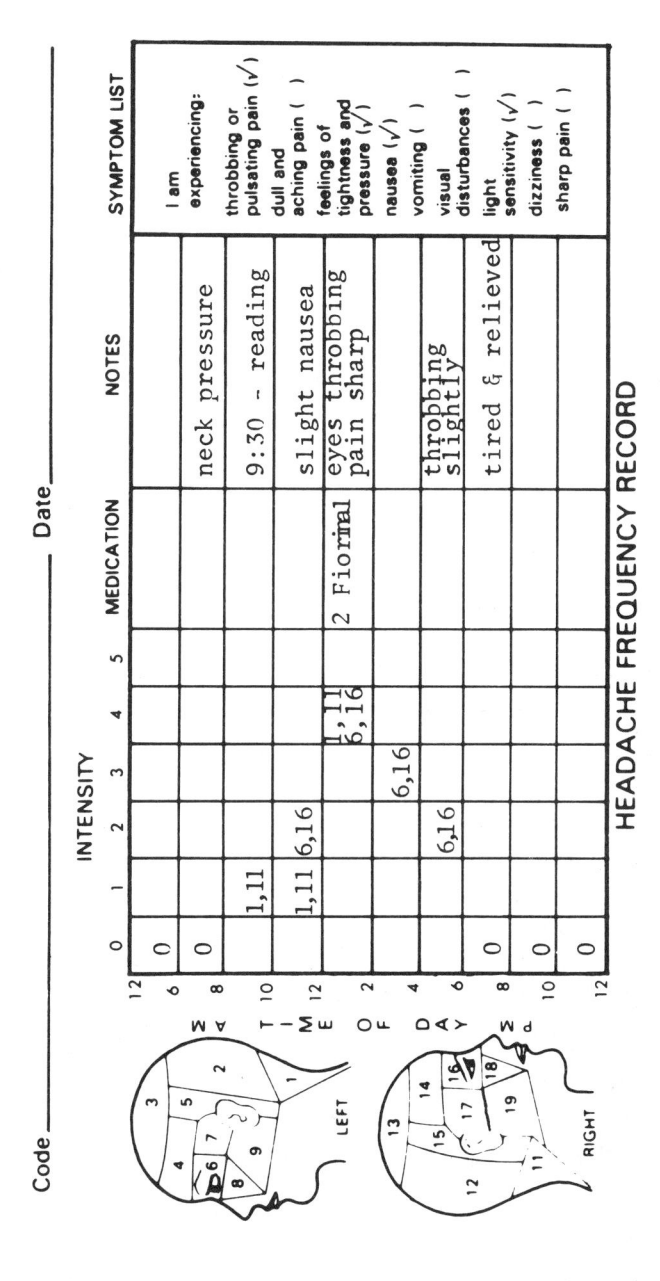

Figure 7.2 Headache frequency record used in rehearsal of self-observation procedure.

records reveal a pattern of headache activity often marked by clocklike regularity serves to strengthen their belief that stress is not the principal cause of their headache attacks. Patients with head pain that develops upon awakening will frequently ask how their disorder could be due to stress given that they slept throughout the night. The therapist simply states that the systems mediating headache attacks (e.g., sustained activity in the musculoskeletal system) may be operative during sleep as well as during the waking state. The patient is directed to discussing what he or she does upon awakening with headache rather than why he or she awakens with headache. The same type of response is used in dealing with other examples of headache attacks that occur in the absence of provocation. In effect, the therapist continually directs the discussion to how the patient deals with headache rather than to why the patient experiences headache.

The therapist reintroduces the notion that headache may be viewed as consisting of a sensory component and a reactive component. The purpose here is to prepare the patient for relaxation training and also to further encourage the reconceptualization process. Usually, there is no problem in getting patients to discuss the sensory component of their headache disorder since they are quite familiar with the degree to which the headache hurts, where it hurts, and so on. This is not always the case with the reactive component. At this point, some patients are unable or unwilling to talk beyond the sensation of pain. However, other patients are more verbal and freely engage in a discussion of the thoughts and feelings that accompany headache attacks. Whether recognized or not, it is too early in the reconceptualization process to press the etiological significance of distress-related cognitions. The therapist simply makes note of their presence and moves on to introducing relaxation training.

Relaxation training is presented as a skill that can be used to deal with the sensory component of headache susceptibility and headache attacks. It is described as a technique that is useful for modifying the physiological component of the disorder, which includes modifying the presence of persistent feelings of tightness and pressure that the patient may experience. The patient is instructed to view relaxation as a skill to be learned with practice. A way to help the patient understand the importance of practice is to use the analogy of learning to drive a car or to ride a bicycle. At first the initial stages of learning are difficult and cumbersome, as they require deliberate and conscious efforts. With practice, however, the skill becomes automatic and requires very little conscious effort. The same process is involved in learning to relax.

The tapes used in the program were developed by Budzynski (1974) and consist of training in passive relaxation as opposed to progressive muscle relaxation. Although progressive muscle relaxation (i.e., training in the alternate tensing and relaxing of different muscle sets) is widely used, this form of relaxation is not always suitable for chronic headache patients. Many patients continuously feel tension, especially in the muscles of the neck and shoulders, and they dislike the additional discomfort generated by the volitional contraction of the muscles. Some patients have reported that the volitional contraction of their muscles produces a state of tension that they cannot immediately release. The Budzynski method of passive relaxation was also specifically designed to be compatible with biofeedback training. The technique employs self-regulatory phrases that are repeated over and over while the listener maintains a focused awareness on the particular body part (e.g., "My right arm is heavy and limp"). Two tapes are used: the first deals with relaxation of the arms and legs, and the second deals with relaxation of the head, neck, and shoulders.

The playing and rehearsal of the first tape is preceded by a brief discussion of the purpose behind the tape and what the patient may expect to happen while listening to the tape. Two reasons are given to the patient for beginning relaxation training with the arms and legs. First, it is much easier to relax the arms and legs than it is to relax the shoulder, neck, and head regions. Second, beginning training with the arms and legs produces a general state of relaxation that enhances the ability to employ passive relaxation to control the muscles of the shoulder, neck, and head regions. The tape begins with relaxation of the right arm, and the patient is encouraged to pay close attention to any sensations that accompany the verbalization of the autogenic phrases. The phrases are explained as verbal aids to help the patient relax, or let go. The patient is instructed to observe whether the arm feels heavy, limp, or whether it tingles or becomes light. Attention then focuses sequentially on the left arm, both arms and hands, and finally the legs. The therapist emphasizes that this form of relaxation is passive and cannot be forced. Another useful suggestion is to advise the patient not to worry if intruding thoughts occur while listening to the tape. The patient should simply let each thought come and go while allowing his or her attention to return to the tape.

Playing the tape is followed by a brief discussion of what the patient experienced while listening to the instructions. The patient is provided with a copy of the tape and is encouraged to practice the technique twice daily during the coming week. The patient is advised not to practice during periods of pain until he or she feels that the relaxation response has been strengthened. The patient is also cautioned not to expect this exercise to have an immediate effect on his or her headache activity.

The third session begins with a review of the patient's experiences during the previous week with the first relaxation tape. The therapist guides the discussion with the following questions: Did your arms and legs become relaxed? What sensations, thoughts, and feelings accompanied the relaxation? Did you find that other thoughts or head pain interfered with your ability to listen to the tape? How often did you practice the tape? Are you able to practice regularly? Is relaxation a pleasurable activity? Most patients report having little difficulty with this tape, and some report the daily practice of the tape to be boring. Some patients report that they did not practice at all because they were too busy with other things. Patients are not admonished for failing to practice; instead, the therapist simply explores the reasons given for the failure. Some patients are disappointed, in spite of the warning, that the relaxation exercise had no effect on their headache activity. Again, the therapist emphasizes that the exercise was not intended to cure the disorder but simply to introduce the patient to relaxation.

The purpose behind the second relaxation tape is described next. It requires the patient to learn to relax the muscles of the head, neck, and shoulder regions. The tape begins by having the listener relax his or her arms and legs, following the procedure of the first tape. The remainder deals with learning to relax the muscles of the jaw, eyes, forehead, neck, shoulders, and temples. The tape ends with a suggestion that the listener may wish to begin practicing a form of cue-controlled relaxation by repeating the phrase "I am calm" whenever he or she feels deeply relaxed. Patients are advised not to expect immediate benefits from using the phrase or to be too concerned about using this form of control. One of the most dramatic positive examples of using the phrase "I am calm" came from a chronic cluster headache sufferer. During the initial playing of the tape in the clinic, he began to develop a cluster attack. He showed increasing signs of pain and distress, until he repeated the phrase to himself. The cluster attack was aborted immediately and completely. This was not an isolated occurrence because he was able to use this phrase to prevent attacks for the next several weeks. The use of cue-controlled relaxation is not emphasized in the present program. If patients find the technique useful, then they are encouraged to use it but only in the context of the overall philosophy of the program. Patients are not left to depend on any specific technique per se unless they incorporate the techniques into altering their overall headache susceptibility.

The fourth session marks the beginning of biofeedback training. The session begins with a discussion of the patient's experiences with the second relaxation tape. The discussion follows the same format that was used for the first tape. Questioning deals with whether or not the patient found time to practice, enjoyed the practice, and improved in relaxing the various muscle sets. Most patients report an improvement in their ability, but at the same time they feel that the skill is far from perfected. Especially difficult are the muscles of the neck and shoulder, which often cannot be relaxed beyond a certain level. They may also complain of interfering thoughts that hamper their efforts during home practice. Patients are encouraged to continue practicing the second tape, and they are told that biofeedback training will be used to help strengthen their ability to relax the muscles of the shoulder, neck, and head regions.

Biofeedback training is introduced with several therapeutic objectives in mind. First, it demonstrates to the patient that the disorder has a physiological component and that his or her thoughts and feelings interact with this component. Second, it facilitates the reconceptualization process by demonstrating to the patient that he or she must take an active role in the treatment process. Third, biofeedback helps the patient discriminate between sensations of relaxation and tension. Finally, biofeedback training allows the patient to focus attention on specific regions that are difficult to control with relaxation training (e.g., shoulder, neck, forehead). Only one feedback modality, EMG feedback, is used in the present program. It may be possible to accomplish the same objectives with other forms of biofeedback, but EMG training is consistent with the severity model as it focuses directly on the musculoskeletal component of the chronic headache syndrome.

Biofeedback training is described to the patient as a technique that will help him or her develop control of muscles of the head, neck, and shoulders. The feedback device is described as a tool that will help the patient become more aware of muscle activity associated with sensations and thoughts and also help him or her develop strategies for reducing the presence of this activity. Changes in muscle activity are fed back in the form of changes in clicks or beeps. Increases in muscle activity are signaled by an increase in the rate of beeps, and decreases are signaled by a decrease in the beep rate.

This relationship is demonstrated by attaching the electrodes to the forehead and asking the patient to clench his or her teeth.

Training starts with the forehead, primarily to ensure that the patient has a positive experience with the procedure. Frontal EMG is easy to manipulate, and it may be that the forehead is also reflective of general tension. The main objective of the first session is to demonstrate to the patient that he or she can voluntarily manipulate the muscle activity in the forehead region. Although encouraged to lower the beep rate as much as possible, the patient is told not to worry about being unsuccessful. The patient is also encouraged to become aware of any thoughts and/or sensations that accompany changes in the feedback signal and, to accomplish this task, the patient is encouraged to experiment on his or her own. It helps to provide the patient with examples of strategies other patients have used. For example, some find that repeating the autogenic phrases from the relaxation tapes is effective. Others use imagery of their own creation such as picturing the muscles in the mind's eye. A cook imagined the muscles turning into melting butter, while a biochemist imagined lactic acid flowing away from the muscles. Still others have used images associated with hypnosis or meditation or simply with being relaxed in some pleasant environment. A final example involves passive awareness, or thinking of nothing. Only a few patients can relate to this strategy, but it serves to demonstrate the diversity of strategies that may be used.

In any one session, the patient receives approximately twenty minutes of actual practice (thirty trials each of forty seconds duration). The patient is never left alone during the period of interaction with the biofeedback machine. The therapist pays careful attention to the patient's performance and makes one or more interruptions during the training trials to discuss with the patient his or her understanding of the task, progress or lack of progress, and strategies being used. If no difficulties are reported and progress is satisfactory, then further interruptions are not made. A problem common to many patients is that they become frustrated after a few trials because they cannot decrease the beep rate. The solution to the difficulty depends on the patient, but sometimes it is because the patient is trying to "force" the signal to change rather than trying to bring about the change through passive relaxation.

The patient is now asked to combine what he or she learned in the present session with what he or she learned during the relaxation training and to continue practicing these skills. Instead of following a "twice daily" format, however, the patient is encouraged to use the skills during the course of his or her daily activities. Thus, the patient is asked to take a few moments during the day to notice the degree and location of bodily tension and then to reduce the tension. This practice might occur while the patient is at work, at home, or while driving or riding to and from work. Patients often do not understand the necessity of incorporating these skills into daily behavior patterns, and the therapist must continually encourage them to do so.

A similar procedure and rationale is followed during the remaining four biofeedback sessions. The therapist continues to strengthen the patient's self-regulatory skill both within the laboratory and within the patient's natural environment. Two of the remaining biofeedback sessions are directed towards training in forehead EMG, and two sessions are directed towards EMG training at other problem sites, if such sites have been reported by the patient (e.g., neck, shoulder). Additional biofeedback sessions may be used if the patient shows evidence that additional sessions might be beneficial. For example, one patient complained following the regular number of sessions that he was agitated with not being able to control the feedback signal. The therapist provided additional sessions, with the suggestion that he pay less attention to the signal and more attention to the thoughts, feelings, and sensations that accompanied changes in the feedback signal. The suggested strategy change was quite successful, as the patient found that eventually he was able to bring about reductions in his frontal EMG level by becoming more aware of his internal state. It is not always easy to determine if a patient will benefit from additional feedback sessions.

Some biofeedback therapists advocate the use of a specified level of EMG activity in deciding upon the number of sessions that a patient should receive. That is, they establish a target level of reduced physiological activity and encourage the patient to reach the target level. Our application of biofeedback departs from this approach. The significance of direct physiological control is de-emphasized in favor of increasing the patient's cognitive control of the processes that regulate his or her disorder. Some patients who exhibit very low levels of physiological activity prior to training are still able to benefit substantially from biofeedback training. It would make little sense to tell these patients that, since the meter indicates they are "relaxed," they must be relaxed. After several training sessions, other patients show no signs of being able to substantially reduce their EMG levels. And yet these same patients often report improvement in their awareness of and ability to control their sensations of tightness and tension. And finally, still other patients are extremely adept at lowering their EMG activity during the training sessions but cannot use this skill in any fashion to modify their headache activity. Because of the tremendous patient variations that occur during biofeedback training, it is recommended that patients not be led to believe that the control of EMG activity is either necessary or sufficient for headache management.

Throughout all the biofeedback training sessions, the therapist continues to assess the degree to which the patient is learning to conceptualize his or her disorder in psychobiological terms. This objective is best attained by not having the patient believe that physiological control during the sessions is the main task at hand. The patient must come to understand the full range of variables (physiological, sensory, affective, cognitive) that control the disorder. The patient is told that what happens between the biofeedback sessions is more important than what happens within the sessions. While the patient works toward mastering control over the sensory component of the disorder, the therapist continues to prepare the groundwork for dealing with the reactive, or cognitive, component. As biofeedback training progresses, the patient continually is encouraged to report the thoughts and feelings that accompany his or her headache attacks. Did the patient experience any distressing thoughts concerning how the headache attacks were interfering with work or social activities? Did the patient wonder if others might view the attacks as an "excuse" to avoid specific duties or responsibilities? With respect to the attack itself, did the patient experience distressing thoughts related to how long the attack would last, how severe the pain might become, and whether medication would work? The therapist also attempts to determine if and how the patient is attempting to cope with the disorder. For example, does the patient try to use his or her relaxation skills prior to and during an attack, and what happens when he or she uses these skills? By adopting this line of questioning, the therapist can increase his or her understanding of the kind of distress-related thoughts that the patient experiences.

During one of the biofeedback sessions, the patient also is given a copy of a headache-assessment questionnaire to complete during the coming week, immediately following his or her next severe headache attack. The questionnaire (Table 7.1) contains a number of items that reflect thoughts and feelings headache sufferers commonly experience during an attack. Although the patient's responses to the questionnaire are not discussed until much later in the program, the questionnaire does serve to have the patient begin to observe the presence of distress-related thoughts and feelings.

Table 7.1 Headache Assessment Questionnaire

Code _____ Date _____ Time _____

Many people report having the following kinds of thoughts and feelings when they notice a headache coming on. We would like to know which of these thoughts/feelings you experience at the onset of a headache attack and to what extent you experience them. Please indicate the extent to which each of the following statements are representative of your thoughts/feelings by circling the appropriate number, ranging from "1" for "not at all representative of my thoughts/feelings" to "4" for "very representative of my thoughts/feelings." For example, if you are feeling very tired and slightly worked up, you would circle "4" for "I feel tired" and "2" for "I feel worked up."

	not at all representative	slightly representative	fairly representative	very representative
1. I feel tired.	1	2	3	4
2. I wonder if I'll have to cancel any plans.	1	2	3	4
3. How am I going to concentrate with this awful headache?	1	2	3	4
4. I am determined not to take any medications.	1	2	3	4
5. I am angry with myself for getting another headache.	1	2	3	4
6. I am afraid of what people think about my headaches.	1	2	3	4
7. I am depressed because I have another headache.	1	2	3	4
8. I am concerned that there is something physically wrong with me.	1	2	3	4
9. I feel totally frustrated because I let myself get another headache.	1	2	3	4
10. I don't want to upset anyone by telling them that I have another headache.	1	2	3	4
11. I wonder what it would be like to never be troubled by headaches.	1	2	3	4

(continued)

Table 7.1 (continued)

	not at all representative	slightly representative	fairly representative	very representative
12. I'm trying to relax and bring this headache under control.	1	2	3	4
13. I am worrying about future plans and commitments.	1	2	3	4
14. I hate to take any medicine, but it looks like I'll have to this time.	1	2	3	4
15. I wish little things wouldn't bother me as much as they do.	1	2	3	4
16. I can tell this one won't be that bad.	1	2	3	4
17. I feel very worked up.	1	2	3	4
18. I feel helpless.	1	2	3	4
19. I am thinking, "Why me? Why do I always get headaches?"	1	2	3	4
20. I wish I could take the time to lie down.	1	2	3	4
21. I can't help feeling angry about what happened before.	1	2	3	4
22. I guess all I can do is wait it out.	1	2	3	4
23. Listening to their chatter makes me feel sick.	1	2	3	4
24. I wonder how long this will last.	1	2	3	4
25. I wonder if they will ever find a sure cure for headaches.	1	2	3	4
26. I am disappointed with myself for getting another headache.	1	2	3	4
27. This headache is driving me crazy.	1	2	3	4
28. I knew this was coming.	1	2	3	4
29. When I stop and think about my headache, it seems to get worse.	1	2	3	4
30. I wish I didn't have to do anything today.	1	2	3	4

Table 7.1 (continued)

		not at all representative	slightly representative	fairly representative	very representative
31.	I feel panic stricken.	1	2	3	4
32.	I wish people would be more considerate.	1	2	3	4
33.	Oh well, now I have a good excuse not to do what I was supposed to do.	1	2	3	4
34.	I'm worried about my family obligations.	1	2	3	4
35.	I can think of nothing other than my pain.	1	2	3	4
36.	I have no patience with others.	1	2	3	4
37.	I feel that I am being punished.	1	2	3	4
38.	When I feel like this, I need comfort from my friends and family.	1	2	3	4
39.	I guess all I can do is wait it out.	1	2	3	4
40.	It's so hard to work with a headache.	1	2	3	4
41.	I wish everyone would be quiet and leave me alone.	1	2	3	4
42.	I feel totally frustrated because I have another headache.	1	2	3	4
43.	I am afraid that my headache will get worse.	1	2	3	4
44.	I'll just have to act as natural as I can.	1	2	3	4
45.	Everyone is getting on my nerves.	1	2	3	4
46.	I am wondering why I'm getting a headache now.	1	2	3	4
47.	I get upset each time I think of what happened before.	1	2	3	4
48.	I feel guilty about having another headache.	1	2	3	4

Following the last biofeedback session, some headache patients are sufficiently improved to discontinue therapy. These patients have altered their susceptibility to headache attacks to the extent that they feel the problem is under control. The predictors of patient improvement following relaxation/biofeedback training are unknown. However, the predictors are not likely to be found from diagnostic parameters associated with the traditional classification system. Patients with the diagnosis of classical migraine, migraine, cluster, and muscle-contraction headaches have shown clinical improvement at the end of biofeedback training. One possibility might be the severity of the disorder as defined by daily headache activity. Patients who experience a large portion of their waking hours in head pain may improve less than patients who experience a small portion of waking hours in pain. Other possible predictors include coping styles and degree of interpersonal support available from significant others. Such variables may logically be expected to influence the patient's ability to understand and incorporate the psychobiological model within his or her daily functioning.

The therapist must use considerable judgment before deciding to terminate therapy with a patient who feels that his or her attacks are now under control. Some patients enthusiastically pronounce themselves "cured" after a few sessions, but at the same time they show signs of not having developed skills beyond the relaxation and biofeedback sessions. They are too dependent on the exercises per se and run the risk that in time the exercises will lose all effectiveness. The risk of relapse is minimized by having the patients return to the clinic after a few weeks of practicing on their own.

Attention-Diversion Training

The ninth session marks the beginning of a shift in emphasis in the treatment program. Beginning with attention-diversion training, the patient is provided with several coping strategies that are presented with the aim of helping reduce the distress generated by recurrent headache attacks. The session begins with a review of what has and has not been accomplished during the previous sessions. The therapist restates the idea that pain consists of both a sensory and a reactive component. The reactive, or cognitive, component is itself divisible into two components. First, there is the amount of attention that is directed towards the headache attack. For example, patients often state that when they have a headache the "whole world becomes a sore head." The pain and misery is so severe that attention cannot be directed toward anything else. The second cognitive component refers to the interpretation of pain or to the train of thoughts and feelings that precede and accompany the pain experience. The interpretive component is demonstrated with examples of self-talk that patients engage in during headache attacks ("Oh no, here we go again"; "I wonder how long this will last"; etc.).

The attention-diversion training begins with a brief discussion of human attention (after Genest, 1977). The patient is told that the process of attention has several properties that are significant for understanding its use in managing headache. First, a person usually only focuses on one thing at a time. This property is demonstrated to the patient by having the patient focus his or her vision on some aspect of the room and observe how other aspects become blurred. Another demonstration involves asking the patient to attend to the therapist's voice and observe how background room noise (e.g., air circulation fan) fades from awareness. The second property is the volitional and immediate nature of attention. A person can influence what he or she wishes to attend to and also can redirect attention from one aspect of his or her environment (internal/external) to another. Finally, it is difficult, if not impossible, to stop paying attention to unpleasant sensations unless one refocuses on other things.

Following the discussion of the nature of attention and its role in pain perception, the patient is given a structured exercise with which to practice controlling his or her attention:

> With your eyes closed, take some time to pay attention to your awareness and notice where it goes. Say to yourself, "Now I am aware of" ... and finish the sentence with what you are focusing on at the moment. Where does your awareness go? ... Are you aware of things outside your body, or sensations inside your skin? ... Now direct your attention to whichever you are least aware of, internal or external, and focus your awareness on this ... To the extent you are occupied with a thought or an image, your awareness of inside and outside reality disappears. Continue experimenting with your awareness and realize that it is like a searchlight. Whatever you focus your attention on is clear, while other objects and events tend to fade from awareness.
>
> If attention is directed to what you hear, you can probably notice different sounds and noises ... and while doing this, you are most likely unaware of the sensations in your hands ... As attention shifts to your hands, awareness of the sounds fades. Your awareness can shift from one thing to another quite rapidly, but you can only fully attend to whatever is in the focus of your awareness at the moment ...
>
> Now notice whatever thoughts or images come into your mind ... Pay attention to these thoughts and be aware of what happens when you try to stop them ... Now try something different. Instead of trying

to stop your thoughts, just focus your attention on your breathing....
Whenever you realize that your attention has wandered back to
thoughts and images, just refocus your awareness on the physical sensations of your breathing... Do not struggle or battle.... just notice
when you are preoccupied with words, images, or sensations, and return your attention to your breathing....

A method of using the attentional exercise is to shift your attention
from internal to external sources of stimulation. You can start with the
sensations in the soles of your feet pressing against the floor and moving slowly up the body... Experience fully the physical sensations of
your body.... Now shift your attention to external stimulation, becoming aware of sounds, noises, and air currents against your face and
neck.... Notice that you must focus your attention on one thing at a
time. Play with your attention.... Move freely back and forth between
internal and external stimulation.

A brief discussion of the attention-diversion exercise follows. Was the patient able to shift attention between external and internal events? Did the patient find that thoughts interfered with his or her ability to make the shift? Although previously aware of the effects of refocusing attention, the majority of patients find the exercise interesting and demonstrate a willingness to practice it further. Patients who experience no difficulties during the rehearsal of the exercise are encouraged to practice the skill at home, both without and with a headache present. With pain present, they are instructed to get involved through ideation, or behavior in some task that directs attention away from the pain. With patients who had difficulties performing the exercise, home practice is directed for periods when they are headache-free.

After a week's home practice, most patients report an improvement in their ability to refocus attention. Some patients now are able to use the technique to significantly reduce the pain they experience during headache attacks. The technique is especially valuable in assisting patients who were previously having difficulties with the relaxation training and biofeedback training components of therapy. These same patients often find that attention-diversion strategies are more compatible with their preferred way of coping than the passive strategies associated with relaxation/biofeedback training. Patients who are still having difficulties are encouraged to maintain their practice. The therapist also continues to work with the patient in identifying situations of attention-diversion that are already occurring in the patient's environment. For example, patients may report that the pain is less when they are involved in housecleaning, reading, working, etc. The patient is made to realize that these are occurrences of attention-diversion and that he or she does have the ability to perform the task. It is important that the therapist use as many examples as the patient provides not only to make the strategy understandable, but also to illustrate the resources already within the patient's command.

Imagery Training

Imagery training is presented in the tenth session. The therapist describes imagery training as a coping strategy that is very similar in nature to attention-diversion. For example, emergency room doctors are known to ask children to imagine they are viewing their favorite television program when an anesthetic cannot be used. People also use imagery in the form of daydreaming to direct their attention away from boring conversationalists (e.g., some college professors). We all often think about something else in order to remove or avoid an unwanted thought or feeling. Thinking about something else is easier than not thinking in order to prevent unpleasant ideation. There are two aspects of the relationship between imagery and headache that are emphasized. First, imagery is a part of all human behavior, including headache attacks; and second, imagery can be used in a constructive fashion to reduce the pain of headache attacks.

To illustrate the relationship between imagery, bodily sensations, and physiological changes, the following two imagery exercises are rehearsed with the patient (both exercises were adapted from Genest, 1977):

Scene I

Try involving yourself in the following image right now, and see how vivid you can make it. Sit back and relax in your chair and listen to this passage. Imagine a pure white plate with a lemon on it, resting on a table. You can clearly see the glossy yellow of the lemon's skin against the whiteness of the china plate.... You can see the texture of the lemon rind, clean and fresh looking.

There is a knife on the table, next to the plate. Imagine that you're picking up the knife. Hold the lemon with one hand, and with the other, using the knife, cut the lemon in two. As the keen edge slices easily into the lemon, the juice runs onto your fingers and the plate. The citrus odor immediately hits your nose: sharp, clean, pungent, delicious, invigorating.

Now pick up one of the lemon halves, with the juice still dripping onto your fingers and the plate. Using the knife cut a wedge from the lemon half, raise the wedge to your mouth and touch your tongue against it gently. Every taste bud in your tongue is drenched with the tangy lemon juice, as your mouth puckers instinctively. A shiver goes up and down your spine and your shoulders shake involuntarily. Now sit back and close your eyes and picture for a moment, the lemon, the cutting, the tasting.

Scene II

Once again, make sure that you are comfortable in your chair and now visualize yourself standing before a large lake, looking out across an expanse of blue water and beyond, to the far shore. Immediately in front of you stretches a small beach and behind you a grassy meadow. The sun is fierce and very hot, bathing the landscape in a shimmering brightness. It is a gorgeous summer day. The sky is pale blue, with great billowy clouds drifting by. The wind is blowing gently, just enough to make the trees sway and make ripples in the grass. Feel the wind on your cheeks. It is a perfect day, and you have it entirely to yourself, with nothing to do, nowhere to go. You have a blanket and you walk off through the meadow. You find a spot, spread the blanket and lie down. It is so warm and quiet. It's such a treat to have the day to yourself to just relax and take it easy. Think about that warm, beautiful day. You walk towards the water, feeling the soft lush grass under your feet. You reach the beach and start across it. Now you can feel the hot sand underfoot. It is almost too hot to stand on, but not quite. It's just very warm and very nice. Now visualize yourself walking into the water slowly, up to your ankles, up to your knees. The water is warm and pleasant. You splash it up around you and feel the wind, now cooling on your wet skin. Look around. You are still all alone. You still have this lovely spot to yourself. Far across the lake you can see a sailboat, tiny in the distance. It is so far away you can just make out the white sail jutting up from the blue water. You take another look around and decide to return to your spot to lie down and enjoy the sun. Across the warm sand to the grass. Now you feel the grass beneath your feet again—deep, soft. You can feel the hot sun warming your skin. It must be 90°, but it is clear and dry. The heat isn't oppressive, it's just nice and warm and comfortable. You lie down on the blanket and feel the deep, soft grass under your head. You're looking up at the sky, seeing great billowy clouds floating by, far, far above. In the distance you can hear the rustle of the water against the shore. You can hear the sound of a bird gently singing in a tree nearby. You even can smell the sweet grass around you. Feel the gentle breeze in your hair and on your skin. You are very comfortable, quite complacent, and totally relaxed. Take a minute or two to sit back, close your eyes, and continue the image on your own.

Most patients have little difficulty becoming involved with these two scenes. While imagining the lemon scene, for example, patients

may begin to salivate and swallow (an observation the therapist uses to illustrate the relationship that exists between thought and physiology). Patients generally find the beach scene to be pleasant, although there are exceptions. One patient reported becoming very uncomfortable during the imagining of this scene. Her imagery was so vivid that she became hot and thirsty. Other patients simply do not like beach scenes, or at least the example provided. Patients are encouraged to view these exercises as examples only. During the coming week, they are instructed to observe the presence and operation of imagery in their daily behaviors, especially in relation to behaviors that precede and accompany their headache attacks. The patient is encouraged to try to identify examples of imagery that can be used to cope with the distress associated with headache attacks. Images generated in this fashion have more meaning to the patients than images generated from a therapist's examples. Quite often the symbolization that is effective for a patient is highly idiosyncratic and unexpected, as illustrated by a patient who felt completely relaxed and at ease while imagining that she was in Las Vegas.

The eleventh session is devoted to a discussion of how attention-diversion and imagery production may be used to control head pain. The patient is given a list (Table 7.2) of the ways in which these two coping strategies may be used. The list of strategies (adapted from Turk, 1978) is offered to determine which coping tactics the patient feels are of potential value. At first glance, some of the strategies might appear to the patient to be of little value. Counting ceiling tiles while experiencing severe head pain might seem futile. However, many patients report that this activity is better than catastrophizing over the pain, misery, and suffering.

Most patients are aware of having engaged in cognitive activities similar to those provided in the list, but they have not considered these activities as representing techniques for coping with pain. The therapist encourages the patient to identify four or five different coping strategies because the patient's dependence on one specific strategy may become difficult, especially during periods of severe pain. By having multiple techniques within his or her command, the patient can alternate between techniques during the course of a headache attack. The patient is asked to strengthen his or her use of these techniques in the absence of pain, in order that the patient's newly-acquired skill is sufficiently strong before the headache attack occurs. Otherwise, the patient may become discouraged and feel that attention-diversion and imagery-production skills are of no present or future use. The patient also is cautioned not to expect the headache attack to simply disappear with the use of these strategies.

Table 7.2 Attention-Diversion and Imagery-Production Strategies

1. Focusing attention on various features of your environment. For example, count ceiling tiles in the doctor's office; study construction of objects present in the room; compare colors and shades of surrounding objects; study various shapes of clouds, trees, houses; detect and analyze various sounds present in the environment.
2. Focusing attention on various thoughts. For example, do mental arithmetic, make a list of all the things you must do over the weekend, think of the words of various songs you recall.
3. Concentrating on a nondemanding task or activity. Engage in some involving activity.
4. Focusing attention on bodily processes or sensations. Recognize that during a headache attack the whole body does not hurt and that attention can be redirected from the painful region to other body sites (e.g., breathing, warmth and comfort in other body regions).
5. Imaginative inattention: using pleasant imagery to attend away from the pain. For example, imagine yourself taking a walk in the forest, or at a party you recently attended during which you had a lot of fun. Recall in detail a movie or play or some other pleasant event you have experienced recently. Repetitive imagery also may be used especially when the pain is severe. For example, imagine yourself sitting on a seashore watching the waves coming one after another, or sitting by a river or a waterfall watching the water flowing by. Imagine the wheel of a water mill slowly turning.
6. Imaginative transformation of the pain sensation: interpreting the pain sensation as something other than headache. For example, imagine having on a tight hat or a headband; imagine the pain sensation as mist slowly dissipating from the painful area; imagine the muscles in the painful area are injected with Novocaine and that they have become numb and insensitive to pain.

Adapted from Turk, 1978

Instead, he or she is encouraged to notice the lessening of pain associated with their use.

A patient's ability to generate vivid images may or may not be predictive of his or her ability to use imagery in therapeutic fashion. Some patients who generate a great number of images during the rehearsal stage cannot manage to use the skill during a headache attack. Other patients who have difficulty producing more than one example of imagery during the training session are able to employ the one image very effectively in coping with pain. A problem with the use of attention-diversion and imagery production is that some patients find their pain increases rather than decreases. Typically, these patients have doubts with respect to the utility of the techniques and often report using the cognitive strategies while simultaneously attending to the pain. There is no easy solution to this difficulty, but the therapist needs to be cognizant of its possible presence.

Thought Management

The final session deals with headache-related thoughts and feelings. By now, patients have acquired considerable understanding of the role that distressing cognitions play in their disorder. For all patients, however, the therapist reviews the idea that the pain experienced during a headache attack depends on more than the physical sensation; it also depends on the amount of attention directed towards the head pain and the patient's interpretation or *appraisal* of the pain. To illustrate the appraisal component of head pain, the therapist uses the patient's responses to the headache assessment questionnaire (Table 7.1) that was administered during the biofeedback sessions.

The patient is encouraged to think of appraisal in terms of self-talk and also to understand that distressing self-talk not only increases the pain experienced but interferes with the ability to employ effective coping strategies. A patient who consistently engages in distressing self-talk ("Why me, why do I always have headaches?" "Damn it, here we go again!") cannot be expected to deal effectively with pain. The therapist suggests that this destructive process can be reversed by intentionally changing what is said to oneself. This can be accomplished by practicing the following procedure. First, the patient must become alert to the presence of distressing thoughts and feelings. Second, the patient must use these distressing cognitions as cues or signals to use positive or constructive self-statements. Finally, the patient must deliberately replace the distressing thoughts with coping-oriented self-statements.

In order to demonstrate the kinds of coping verbalizations that may be used, the patient is provided with a list of self-statements (Turk, 1978) to be used during different stages of the headache attack. The statements are presented as examples only and not as statements that must be adopted verbatim. See Table 7.3.

Once these statements have been rehearsed, the therapist assesses the patient's overall position with respect to the various phases of the program. If there are still signs of confusion in the patient, the therapist might wish to add a final session in which he or she rehearses and models all aspects of the program. Usually, however, the patient feels confident that he or she now has a better

Table 7.3 Self-Statements for Coping with Headache

A. The beginning headache
   (1) What is it I have to do? (View the developing pain as a problem that you can do something about.)
   (2) I can develop a plan to deal with it. (Prepare oneself by making a plan or mental outline of how you will deal with the sensations when they arise.)
   (3) Just think about what I have to do. (Focus on what the situation requires.)
   (4) Think of the things that I can use to help cope. (Review all the strategies that you know and that may be helpful.)
   (5) Don't worry; worrying won't help anything. (Use any anxiety or worry as a cue to remind you to focus on what you have to do.)
   (6) Remember, I can shift my attention to anything I want to. (Reassure yourself about your ability to employ various coping strategies.)
   (7) When I use mental imagery, I'll see how vivid I can make the scene. (Review various aspects of the different images and strategies that can be used.)
B. Confronting the pain
   (1) I can deal with the pain as a challenge. (View the pain as a challenge rather than as a disaster.)
   (2) One step at a time, I can handle the pain. (Don't do everything at once and don't be overwhelmed; rather, use each of the skills you have learned.)
   (3) Just relax, breathe deeply, and use one of the strategies.
   (4) I won't think about the pain, just about what I have to do. (Focus your attention on the task at hand and what you can do right now to help you cope.)
   (5) I'm feeling tense; that can be an ally, a cue to switch strategies, and to take some slow deep breaths.
   (6) Remember, I can switch back to some strategies that I used before.
C. Coping with thoughts and feelings at critical moments (when you notice that the intensity of the pain seems to be increasing or you think that you can't go on any more). Self-instructions or statements that can be made at this phase include:
   (1) When I feel pain, I just pause and keep focusing on what I have to do. (Keep in mind the task at hand and what you have to do.)
   (2) (Don't try to eliminate the pain totally, just keep it manageable. Remember, you expected to detect some intense stimulation, but don't overreact and make things worse.)
   (3) I knew the sensations would rise; I will just keep them under control. (Don't magnify the intensity of the sensations you experience.)
   (4) Remember, there are lots of things I can do; I can keep things under control. (You have been taught a number of different strategies that will help you keep the intense stimulation under control.)

(5) Things are going pretty bad; I can't take any more—just pause; don't make things worse. I'll review my plan of strategies to see what I can switch to. (Sometimes you may have unpleasant thoughts or feelings; use those as cues to review the strategies available for you to use.)
(6) My head feels terrible; things are falling apart; I better stop—relax. I can focus my attention on something else; keep things under control. (If you find yourself focusing on unpleasant sensations or thoughts, remember you can choose what you will focus your attention upon.)

D. (Self-reflection and positive self-statements. Throughout the three phases outlined above, you might evaluate your performance. For example, how am I doing, that worked pretty well, etc. Remember, people frequently criticize themselves but rarely praise their behavior. Throughout a stressful situation, evaluate how you are doing. If you think you should be doing better, you can use that as a cue to try different strategies. If you are doing well, you should give yourself a "pat on the back.") Self-reflective statements that might be used include:
(1) I'm doing pretty well; it's not as hard as I thought.
(2) I'm doing better all the time.
(3) I won't let negative thoughts interfere with my plan.
(4) I knew I could handle it; I'm doing pretty well.

Adapted from Turk, 1978

understanding of the disorder and has a number of skills that can be practiced and improved upon in future dealings with headache attacks. Quite often this new understanding involves nothing more than an awareness that negative self-talk does occur during headache attacks. However, the awareness becomes a powerful tool that the patient can use to "short-circuit" distress reactions and decrease the severity and duration of attacks. Furthermore, this awareness also encompasses other controlling aspects of the disorder, resulting in a significant reduction in the frequency of attacks.

The degree of self-control achieved by patients by the end of the program represents only a beginning in the long-term management of headache. Many patients continue strengthening their new skills to the point that headache no longer interferes with their lives. This represents a remarkable outcome for patients who, after years of undergoing repeated medical examinations and of consuming countless medications, are able to resume normal functioning with the confidence that they are in control. Although often dramatic and exciting, the successful outcomes should not make us lose sight of the fact that additional theoretical and clinical work needs to be done. There are still too many patients who do not improve sufficiently or who do not improve at all. Clearly, this program represents only a beginning, albeit a very positive beginning.

Conclusion

The material contained in this book was presented with the aim of fostering a new approach to the study of chronic headache sufferers. This was accomplished by examining the various aspects of headache knowledge within the framework of a psychobiological model of headache. By adopting this approach, it was possible to view the different dimensions of headache research (genetic, biochemical, physiological, psychological) within a unitary framework and thereby develop the beginnings of a truly holistic understanding of headache patients and their symptoms. Although the model depends heavily for its support on existing knowledge of headache mechanisms, it also requires that theoreticians, researchers, and clinicians begin to appreciate the transactions that take place between the various components of the headache syndrome.

From the psychobiological perspective, all headache sufferers, regardless of presenting symptomatology, are assumed to share a similar predisposition for headache attacks. Rather than being genetically determined, the predisposition is viewed as a global property of the patient, which becomes more involved and encompassing as a result of the failure to cope with less severe headache attacks. Headache susceptibility is a property of the patient that emerges from his or her continued experiences with the disorder and thus involves psychological as well as physiological processes. The predisposition is believed to mediate headache attacks that are precipitated by known events (stress, foodstuffs, weather changes) as well as headaches that seem to occur spontaneously. In chronic headache sufferers, the predisposition is viewed as operating relatively autonomously from the events known to trigger headache attacks in occasional headache sufferers.

A significant aspect of the model concerns the nature of symptoms experienced by headache sufferers, both in clinical instances and in the general population. After examining the data, it was concluded that there is no empirical basis to the belief that muscle-contraction and migraine symptoms occur in the form of relatively pure symptom clusters. Observations based on clinical patients, children with problem headache, and occasional headache sufferers indicated that virtually all headache sufferers experience symptom configurations that, although often highly idiosyncratic, are based on some configuration of both muscle-contraction and migraine symptoms. Although the number of configurations may prove to be finite, it is advantageous to view these symptom configurations as occurring along a continuum of headache severity.

The precise delineation of how chronic headache disorders develop requires longitudinal investigation. However, it is significant that children with varying degrees of problem headache show no tendency to exhibit pure cultures of muscle-contraction and migraine symptoms. To the contrary, they exhibit patterns of headache symptoms and headache activity that are entirely consistent with a severity approach. For, as their disorder increases in severity, they also begin to experience a greater number of muscle-contraction and migraine headache symptoms. Children with the most severe headache activity also show signs of having progressed to a stage of chronicity comparable to that observed in adults, in that they also experience recurrent headache attacks in the absence of precipitating physical and/or psychological events.

Another significant aspect of the severity approach concerns the emphasis placed on the cognitive component of the chronic headache syndrome. It was proposed that recurrent headache attacks are accompanied by the development of distress-related beliefs, thoughts, and feelings that influence and are influenced by the pain experienced. It was proposed that psychological variables be viewed as components rather than as causes of the chronic headache syndrome. Depression, anxiety, and feelings of helplessness and hopelessness are not seen as reflecting the root causes of the problem, but rather they are seen as a significant cognitive component of the headache syndrome. This theoretical position represents a departure from the traditional study of psychological factors in headache, but it is a departure that has already increased our understanding of headache patients. It is encouraging that this change in emphasis, from antecedents to components, when implemented in therapy, is associated with clinically significant reductions in headache activity.

The future of the psychobiological/severity model appears promising. It accounts very well for the current body of headache knowledge that, without the model, lacks cohesiveness and direction. Although presenting a host of new theoretical and clinical challenges, it is anticipated that the model will become increasingly attractive as researchers and clinicians are required by their empirical and clinical observations to invoke psychobiological variables for understanding and treating headache patients. Headache sufferers will be the real beneficiaries of the approach because they become active participants in the development of the model. In fact one of the most rewarding aspects of working with this framework is that it is consistent with the experiences of headache sufferers themselves. Like therapy, theory development works best when all the participants work towards a shared conceptualization of the problem.

References

Ad Hoc Committee on Classification of Headache. Classification of headache. *Journal of the American Medical Association,* 1962, *179,* 717–718.

Allan, W. The inheritance of migraine. *Archives of Internal Medicine,* 1928, *42,* 590–599.

Anderson, C. D., & Franks, R. D. Migraine and tension headache: Is there a physiological difference? *Headache,* 1981, *21,* 63–71.

Anderson, J. A. D., Basker, M. A., & Dalton, R. Migraine and hypnotherapy. *The International Journal of Clinical and Experimental Hypnosis,* 1975, *23,* 48–58.

Andersson, P. G. Ergotamine headache. *Headache,* 1975, *15,* 118–121.

Andrasik, F., Blanchard, E. B., Arena, J. G., Teders, S. J., Teevan, R. C., & Rodichok, L. D. *Psychological functioning in headache sufferers.* Unpublished manuscript, 1981.

Andrasik, F., & Holroyd, K. A. A test of specific and nonspecific effects in the biofeedback treatment of tension headache. *Journal of Consulting and Clinical Psychology,* 1980, *48,* 575–586.

Andreychuk, T., & Skriver, C. Hypnosis and biofeedback in the treatment of migraine headache. *International Journal of Clinical and Experimental Hypnosis,* 1975, *23,* 172–183.

Ansel, E. L. A simple exercise to enhance response to hypnotherapy for migraine headache. *The International Journal of Clinical and Experimental Hypnosis,* 1977, *25,* 68–71.

Appenzeller, O., Davison, K., & Marshall, J. Reflex vasomotor abnormalities in the hands of migrainous subjects. *Journal of Neurology, Neurosurgery and Psychiatry,* 1963, *26,* 447–450.

Bakal, D. A. *Psychology and medicine: Psychobiological dimensions of health and illness.* New York: Springer, 1979.

Bakal, D. A., Demjen, S., & Kaganov, J. A. Cognitive behavioral treatment of chronic headache. *Headache,* 1981, *21,* 81–86.

Bakal, D. A., & Kaganov, J. A. A simple method for self-observation of headache frequency, intensity, and location. *Headache,* 1976, *16,* 123–124.

Bakal, D. A., & Kaganov, J. A. Muscle contraction and migraine headache: Psychophysiologic comparison. *Headache,* 1977, *17,* 208–214.

Bakal, D. A., & Kaganov, J. A. Symptom characteristics of chronic and nonchronic headache sufferers. *Headache,* 1979, *19,* 285–289.

Barber, T. X., Spanos, N. P., & Chaves, J. F. *Hypnotism, imagination, and human potentialities.* New York: Pergamon, 1974.

Basmajian, J. V. Facts vs. myths in EMG biofeedback. *Biofeedback and Self-regulation,* 1976, *1,* 369–371.

Beaty, E. T., & Haynes, S. N. Behavioral intervention with muscle-contraction headache: A review. *Psychosomatic Medicine,* 1979, *41,* 165–180.

Beecher, H. K. *Measurement of subjective responses: Quantitative effects of drugs.* New York: Oxford, 1959.

Beecher, H. K. Quantification of the subjective pain experience. In M. Weisenberg (Ed.), *Pain: Clinical and experimental perspectives.* Saint Louis: Mosby, 1975.

Bibace, R., & Walsh, M. E. *The development of children's concepts of health and illness.* Paper presented at the meeting of the American Psychological Association, San Francisco, August, 1977.

Bille, B. O. Migraine in school children. *Acta Paediatrica,* 1962, *51,* Suppl. 136, 1–151.

Blanchard, E. B., Andrasik, F., Arena, J. G., & Teders, S. J. Variation in meaning of pain descriptors for different headache types as revealed by psychophysical scaling. *Headache,* in press.

Blanchard, E. B., Theobald, D. E., Williamson, D. A., Silver, B. V., & Grown, D. A. Temperature biofeedback in the treatment of migraine headaches. *Archives of General Psychiatry,* 1978, *35,* 581–588.

Blumenthal, L. S. Hypnotherapy of headache. *Headache,* 1963, *2,* 197–202.

Bruyn, G. W. The biochemistry of migraine. *Headache,* 1980, *20,* 234–246.

Budzynski, T. H. *Relaxation training program.* New York: Bio Monitoring Applications Inc., 1974.

Budzynski, T., Stoyva, J., & Adler, C. Feedback-induced muscle relaxation: Application to tension headache. *Journal of Behavior Therapy and Experimental Psychiatry,* 1970, *1,* 205–211.

Cameron, R. The clinical implementation of behavior change techniques: A cognitively oriented conceptualization of therapeutic "compliance" and "resistance." In J. P. Foreyt & D. P. Rathjen (Eds.), *Cognitive behavior therapy: Research and application.* New York: Plenum, 1978.

Cohen, F., & Lazarus, R. S. Coping with the stresses of illness. In G. C. Stone, F. Cohen, & N. E. Adler (Eds.), *Health psychology.* San Francisco: Jossey-Bass, 1980.

References

Cohen, M. J., & Johnson, H. J. Effects of intensity and the signal value of stimuli on the orienting and defensive responses. *Journal of Experimental Psychology*, 1971, *88*, 286–288.

Cohen, M. J., McArthur, D. L., & Rickles, W. Comparison of four biofeedback treatments for migraine headache: Physiological and headache variables. *Psychosomatic Medicine*, 1980, *42*, 463–480.

Couch, J. R., & Hassanein, R. S. Amitriptyline in migraine prophylaxis. *Archives of Neurology*, 1979, *36*, 695–699.

Couch, J. R., Ziegler, D. K., & Hassanein, R. S. Evaluation of the relationship between migraine headache and depression. *Headache*, 1975, *15*, 41–50.

Coyne, J. C., & Lazarus, R. S. Cognitive style, stress perception, and coping. In I. L. Kutash & L. B. Schlesinger (Eds.), *Handbook on stress and anxiety*. San Francisco: Jossey-Bass, 1980.

Curran, D. A., Hinterberger, H., & Lance, J. W. Total plasma serotonin, 5-hydroxy-indoleacetic acid and p-hydroxy-m-methoxymandelic acid excretion in normal and migrainous subjects. *Brain*, 1965, *88*, 997–1010.

Dalessio, D. J. Mechanisms and biochemistry of headache. *Postgraduate Medicine*, 1974, *56*, 55–62.

Dalessio, D. J. Migraine. In D. J. Dalessio (Ed.), *Wolff's headache and other head pain* (4th ed.). New York: Oxford University Press, 1980. (a)

Dalessio, D. J. Migraine therapy. In D. J. Dalessio (Ed.), *Wolff's headache and other head pain* (4th ed.). New York: Oxford University Press, 1980. (b)

Dalsgaard-Nielsen, T. Migraine and heredity. *Acta Neurologica Scandinavica*, 1965, *41*, 287–300.

Dalton, K. Progesterone suppositories and pessaries in the treatment of menstrual migraine. *Headache*, 1973, *12*, 151–159.

Demjen, S., & Bakal, D. Illness behavior and chronic headache. *Pain*, 1981, *10*, 221–229.

De Piano, F. A., & Salzberg, H. C. Clinical applications of hypnosis to three psychosomatic disorders. *Psychological Bulletin*, 1979, *86*, 1223–1235.

Deubner, D. C. An epidemiologic study of migraine and headache in 10–20 year olds. *Headache*, 1977, *17*, 173–180.

Dexter, J. D., Roberts, J., & Byer, J. A. The five hour glucose tolerance test and effect of low sucrose diet in migraine. *Headache*, 1978, *18*, 91–94.

Diamond, S., & Dalessio, D. J. *The practicing physician's approach to headache* (2nd ed.). Baltimore: Williams & Wilkins, 1978.

Edmeads, J. Vascular headaches and the cranial circulation—another look. *Headache*, 1979, *19*, 127–132.

Elmore, A. M., & Tursky, B. A comparison of two psychophysiological approaches to the treatment of migraine. *Headache*, 1981, *21*, 93–101.

Engel, G. L. The need for a new medical model: A challenge for biomedicine. *Science*, 1977, *196*, 129–136.

Evans, F. J. The placebo response in pain reduction. In J. J. Bonica (Ed.),

Advances in neurology (Vol. 4). *International Symposium on Pain.* New York: Raven Press, 1974.

Frank, R. T. The hormonal causes of premenstrual tension. *Archives of Neurology and Psychiatry,* 1931, *26,* 1053–1057.

Frankl, V. E. Reductionism and nihilism. In A. Koestler & J. R. Smythies (Eds.), *Beyond reductionism.* London: Hutchinson, 1969.

French, E. B., Lassers, B. W., & Desai, M. G. Reflex vasomotor responses in the hands of migrainous subjects. *Journal of Neurology, Neurosurgery and Psychiatry,* 1967, *30,* 276–278.

Friar, L. R., & Beatty, J. Migraine: Management by trained control of vasoconstriction. *Journal of Consulting and Clinical Psychology,* 1976, *44,* 46–53.

Friedman, A. P., von Storch, T. J. C., & Merritt, H. H. Migraine and tension headaches: A clinical study of two thousand cases. *Neurology,* 1954, *4,* 773–788.

Genest, M. *A bibliotherapy manual for the control of experimental pain.* Unpublished manuscript, University of Waterloo, 1977.

Genest, M., & Turk, D. C. A proposed model for group therapy with pain patients. In D. Upper & S. M. Ross (Eds.), *Behavioral group therapy: An annual review.* Research Press, 1979.

Goodell, H., Lewontin, R., & Wolff, H. G. Familial occurrence of migraine headache. *Archives of Neurology and Psychiatry,* 1954, *72,* 325–334.

Graham, J. R. Migraine headache: Diagnosis and management. *Headache,* 1979, *19,* 133–141.

Graham, J. R., & Wolff, H. G. Mechanisms of migraine headache and action of ergotamine tartrate. *Archives of Neurology and Psychiatry,* 1938, *39,* 737–763.

Grant, E. C. G. Food allergies and migraine. *Lancet,* 1979, *1,* 966–968.

Green, J. E. Migraine abroad: A survey of migraine in England, 1975–1976. *Headache,* 1977, *17,* 67–68.

Greenblatt, D. J., & Shader, R. I. *Benzodiazepines in clinical practice.* New York: Raven Press, 1974.

Hakkarainen, H., Quiding, H., & Stockman, O. Mild analgesics as an alternative to ergotamine in migraine. A comparative trial with acetylsalicylic acid, ergotamine tartrate, and a dextropropoxyphene compound. *The Journal of Clinical Pharmacology,* 1980, *20,* 590–595.

Halpern, L. M. *The role of drugs in treating chronic pain.* New York: Bio Monitoring Applications, 1978.

Harding, H. C. Hypnosis and migraine or vice versa. *Northwest Medicine,* 1961, *60,* 168–172.

Harper, R. G., & Steger, J. C. Psychological correlates of frontalis EMG and pain in tension headache. *Headache,* 1978, *18,* 215–218.

Harrison, R. H. Psychological testing in headache: A review. *Headache,* 1975, *14,* 177–185.

References

Henryk-Gutt, R., & Rees, W. L. Psychological aspects of migraine. *Journal of Psychosomatic Research*, 1973, *17*, 141–153.

Hilgard, E. R. The alleviation of pain by hypnosis. *Pain*, 1975, *1*, 213–231.

Hockaday, J. M., MacMillan, A. L., & Whitty, C. W. M. Vasomotor reflex response in idiopathic and hormone dependent migraine. *Lancet*, 1967, *1*, 1023–1026.

Holmes, T. H., & Rahe, R. H. The Social Readjustment Rating Scale. *Journal of Psychosomatic Research*, 1967, *11*, 213–218.

Holroyd, K. A. A cognitive-behavioral approach to recurrent tension and migraine headache. In P. C. Kendall (Ed.), *Advances in cognitive-behavioral research and therapy*. New York: Academic Press, in press.

Holroyd, K. A., & Andrasik, F. Coping and the self-control of chronic tension headache. *Journal of Consulting and Clinical Psychology*, 1978, *46*, 1036–1045.

Holroyd, K. A., Andrasik, F., & Westbrook, T. Cognitive control of tension headache. *Cognitive Therapy and Research*, 1977, *1*, 121–133.

Hunter, M., & Philips, C. The experience of headache—an assessment of the qualities of tension headache pain. *Pain*, 1981, *10*, 209–219.

Ingvar, D. H. Pain in the brain—and migraine. *Hemicrania*, 1976, 7, 2–6.

Jay, G. W., & Tomasi, L. G. Pediatric headaches: A one year retrospective analysis. *Headache*, 1981, *21*, 5–9.

Jessup, B. The role of diet in migraine: Conditioned taste aversion. *Headache*, 1978, *18*, 229. (Letter to the editor)

Jessup, B. A., Neufeld, R. W. J., & Merskey, H. Biofeedback therapy for headache and other pain: An evaluative review. *Pain*, 1979, 7, 225–270.

Joffe, R., Bakal, D. A., & Kaganov, J. A. *A self-observation study of headache symptoms experienced by children*. *Headache*, (in press).

Kaganov, J. *The distribution of headache symptoms: An epidemiological study*. Unpublished doctoral dissertation. University of Calgary, Dec. 1980.

Kaganov, J. A., Bakal, D. A., & Dunn, B. E. The differential contribution of muscle contraction and migraine symptoms to problem headache in the general population. *Headache*, 1981, *21*, 157–163.

Kudrow, L. Thermographic and doppler flow asymmetry in cluster headache. *Headache*, 1979, *19*, 204–208. (a)

Kudrow, L. Cluster headache: Diagnosis and management. *Headache*, 1979, *19*, 142–150. (b)

Kudrow, L., & Sutkus, B. J. MMPI pattern specificity in primary headache disorders. *Headache*, 1979, *19*, 18–24.

Kunkel, R. S. Evaluating the headache patient: History and workup. *Headache*, 1979, *19*, 122–126.

Lance, J. W. *Mechanism and management of headache* (2nd ed.). London: Butterworth, 1973.

Legewie, H. Clinical implications of biofeedback. In J. Beatty & H. Legewie (Eds.), *Biofeedback and behavior*. New York: Plenum, 1977.

Lennox, W. G. *Epilepsy and related disorders* (Vol. 1). Boston: Little, Brown, 1960.

Levendusky, P., & Pankratz, L. Self-control techniques as an alternative to pain medication. *Journal of Abnormal Psychology*, 1975, *84*, 165–168.

Liebeskind, J. C., & Paul, L. A. Psychological and physiological mechanisms of pain. *Annual Review of Psychology*, 1977, *28*, 41–60.

Lucas, R. N. Migraine in twins. *Journal of Psychosomatic Research*, 1977, *20*, 147–156.

Mahoney, M. J. Psychotherapy and the structure of personal revolutions. In M. J. Mahoney (Ed.), *Psychotherapy process: Current issues and future directions*. New York: Plenum, 1980.

Marcussen, R. M., & Wolff, H. G. A formulation of the dynamics of the migraine attack. *Psychosomatic Medicine*, 1949, *11*, 251–256.

Markush, R. E., Karp, H. R., Heyman, A., & O'Fallon, W. M. Epidemiologic study of migraine symptoms in young women. *Neurology*, 1975, *25*, 430–435.

Martin, M. J. Muscle contraction headache. *Psychosomatics*, 1972, *13*, 16–19.

Mason, J. W. A historical view of the stress field (Part II). *Journal of Human Stress*, 1975, *1*, 22–36.

Mathew, N. T., Hrastnik, F., & Meyer, J. S. Regional cerebral blood flow in the diagnosis of vascular headache. *Headache*, 1976, *15*, 252–260.

Mechanic, D. The concept of illness behavior. *Journal of Chronic Disease*, 1962, *15*, 189–195.

Medina, J. L., & Diamond, S. The role of diet in migraine. *Headache*, 1978, *18*, 31–34.

Meichenbaum, D. Cognitive factors in biofeedback therapy. *Biofeedback and Self-Regulation*, 1976, *1*, 201–216.

Meichenbaum, D. *Cognitive behavior modification: An integrative approach*. New York: Plenum, 1978.

Melzack, R. *The puzzle of pain*. Harmondsworth: Penguin, 1973.

Melzack, R. The McGill Pain Questionnaire: Major properties and scoring methods. *Pain*, 1975, *1*, 277–299.

Mitchell, K. R., & White, R. G. Behavioral self-management: An application to the problem of migraine headaches. *Behavior Therapy*, 1977, *8*, 213–221.

Moffett, A. M., Swash, M., & Scott, D. F. Effect of chocolate in migraine: A double-blind study. *Journal of Neurology, Neurosurgery, and Psychiatry*, 1974, *37*, 445–448.

Morley, S. Migraine: A generalized vasomotor dysfunction? A critical review of evidence. *Headache*, 1977, *17*, 71–74.

Nattero, G., Bisbocci, D., & Ceresa, F. Sex hormones, prolactin levels, osmolarity and electrolyte patterns in menstrual migraine—Relationship with fluid retention. *Headache,* 1979, *19,* 25–30.

O'Brien, M. D. Cerebral blood changes in migraine. *Headache,* 1971, *10,* 139–143.

Olesen, J. Some clinical features of the acute migraine attack. An analysis of 750 patients. *Headache,* 1978, *18,* 268–271.

Olesen, J., Aebelholt, A., & Veilis, B. The Copenhagen Acute Headache Clinic: Organization, patient material and treatment results. *Headache,* 1979, *19,* 223–227.

Ostfeld, A. M., & Wolff, H. G. Identification, mechanisms and management of the migraine syndrome. *Medical Clinics of North America,* 1958, *42,* 1497–1509.

Otis, S. M., Smith, R. A., Kroll, A. D., Krasny, S. E., Seltzer, K. A., & Dalessio, D. J. Vasospasm and vascular headaches: Selective vasoconstriction in the carotid vascular system measured by the Doppler Ophthalmic Method in migraineurs. *Headache,* 1979, *19,* 200–203.

Parnell, P., & Cooperstock, R. Tranquilizers and mood elevators in the treatment of migraine: An analysis of the Migraine Foundation questionnaire. *Headache,* 1979, *19,* 78–89.

Pearce, J. P. Migraine: A psychosomatic disorder. *Headache,* 1977, *17,* 125–128.

Philips, C. Headache and personality. *Journal of Psychosomatic Research,* 1976, *20,* 535–542.

Philips, C. The modification of tension headache pain using EMG biofeedback. *Behavior Research and Therapy,* 1977, *15,* 119–129.

Philips, C. Tension headache: Theoretical problems. *Behavior Research and Therapy,* 1978, *16,* 249–261.

Pilowsky, I., & Spence, N. D. Patterns of illness behavior in patients with intractable pain. *Journal of Psychosomatic Research,* 1975, *19,* 279–287.

Pózniak-Patewicz, E. "Cephalic" spasm of head and neck muscles. *Headache,* 1976, *15,* 261–266.

Price, K. P., & Clarke, L. K. Classical conditioning of digital pulse volume in migraineurs and normal controls. *Headache,* 1979, *19,* 328–332.

Raskin, N. H., & Appenzeller, O. *Headache.* Philadelphia: Saunders, 1980.

Rogado, A., Harrison, R. H., & Graham, J. R. *Personality profiles in cluster headache, migraine, and normal controls.* Paper presented at the 10th International Congress of World Federation of Neurology, Kyoto, Japan, September, 1973.

Rolf, L. H., Wiele, G., & Brune, G. G. 5-Hydroxytryptamine in platelets of patients with muscle contraction headache. *Headache,* 1981, *21,* 10–11.

Ruble, D. N., & Brooks-Gunn, J. Menstrual symptoms: A social cognitive analysis. *Journal of Behavioral Medicine,* 1979, *2,* 171–194.

Sacks, O. *Migraine: Evolution of a common disorder.* London: Pan Books, 1981.

Sakai, F., & Meyer, J. S. Regional cerebral hemodynamics during migraine and cluster headaches measured by the ^{133}Xe inhalation method. *Headache,* 1978, *18,* 122–132.

Sargent, J. D., Green, E. E., & Walters, E. D. The use of autogenic training in a pilot study of migraine and tension headaches. *Headache,* 1972, *12,* 120–124.

Schwartz, G. The brain as a health care system. In G. C. Stone, F. Cohen, & N. E. Adler (Eds.), *Health psychology.* San Francisco: Jossey-Bass, 1980.

Selby, G., & Lance, J. W. Observations on 500 cases of migraine and allied vascular headache. *Journal of Neurology, Neurosurgery, and Psychiatry,* 1960, *23,* 23–32.

Selye, H. *The stress of life.* New York: McGraw-Hill, 1956.

Shapiro, A. K., & Morris, L. A. The placebo effect in medical and psychological therapies. In S. L. Garfield & A. E. Bergin (Eds.), *Handbook of psychotherapy and behavior change: An empirical analysis* (2nd ed.). New York: Wiley & Sons, 1978.

Sicuteri, F. Headache: Disruption of pain modulation. In J. J. Bonica & D. Albe-Fessard (Eds.), *Advances in pain research and therapy* (Vol. 1). New York: Raven Press, 1976.

Silver, B. V., & Blanchard, E. B. Biofeedback and relaxation training in the treatment of psychophysiological disorders: Or are the machines really necessary? *Journal of Behavioral Medicine,* 1978, *1,* 217–239.

Simard, D., & Paulson, O. B. Cerebral vasomotor paralysis during migraine attack. *Archives of Neurology,* 1973, *29,* 207–209.

Sjaastad, O. The significance of blood serotonin levels in migraine. *Acta Neurologica Scandinavica,* 1975, *51,* 200–210.

Skinhoj, E., & Paulson, O. B. Regional blood flow in internal carotid distribution during migraine attack. *British Medical Journal,* 1969, *3,* 569–570.

Smith, C. H. Recurrent vomiting in children. *Journal of Pediatrics,* 1937, *10,* 719–742.

Sokolov, Y. N. *Perception and the conditioned reflex.* New York: Macmillan, 1963.

Sovak, M., Kunzel, M., Sternbach, R. A., & Dalessio, D. J. Is volitional manipulation of hemodynamics a valid rationale for biofeedback therapy of migraine? *Headache,* 1978, *18,* 197–202.

Sovak, M., Kunzel, M., Sternbach, R. A., & Dalessio, D. J. Mechanism of the biofeedback therapy of migraine: Volitional manipulation of the psychophysiological background. *Headache,* 1981, *21,* 89–92.

Spanos, N. P., Radtke-Bodorik, H. L., Ferguson, J. D., & Jones, B. The effects of hypnotic susceptibility, suggestions for analgesia, and the utilization of cognitive strategies on the reduction of pain. *Journal of Abnormal Psychology*, 1979, *88*, 282-292.

Sternbach, R. A. *Pain patients: Traits and treatment.* New York: Academic Press, 1974.

Swanson, D. W., Swenson, W. M., Maruta, T., & McPhee, M. C. Program for managing chronic pain. 1. Program description and characteristics of patients. *Mayo Clinic Proceedings*, 1976, *51*, 401-408.

Tfelt-Hansen, P., Lous, I., & Olesen, J. Prevalence and significance of muscle tenderness during common migraine attacks. *Headache*, 1981, *21*, 49-54.

Thompson, J. K., Haber, J. D., Figueroa, J. L., & Adams, H. E. A replication and generalization of the "Psychobiological" model of headache. *Headache*, 1980, *20*, 199-203.

Tunis, M. M., & Wolff, H. G. Studies on headache: Cranial artery vasoconstriction and muscle contraction headache. *Archives of Neurology and Psychiatry*, 1954, *71*, 425-434.

Turin, A., & Johnson, W. G. Biofeedback therapy for migraine headaches. *Archives of General Psychiatry*, 1976, *33*, 577-579.

Turk, D. C. Cognitive behavioral techniques in the management of pain. In J. P. Foreyt & D. P. Rathjen (Eds.), *Cognitive behavior therapy: Research and application.* New York: Plenum, 1978.

Turk, D. C. *Cognitive therapy for pain.* New York: BMA Audio Cassettes, 1980.

Turk, D. C., Meichenbaum, D. H., & Berman, W. H. Application of biofeedback for the regulation of pain: A critical review. *Psychological Bulletin*, 1979, *86*, 1322-1338.

Tursky, B. The development of a pain perception profile: A psychophysical approach. In M. Weisenberg & B. Tursky (Eds.), *Pain: New perspectives in therapy and research.* New York: Plenum, 1976.

Waters, W. E. Migraine: Intelligence, social class and familial prevalence. *British Medical Journal*, 1971, *2*, 77-78.

Waters, W. E. The epidemiological enigma of migraine. *International Journal of Epidemiology*, 1973, *2*, 189-194.

Waters, W. E. The Pontypridd headache survey. *Headache*, 1974, *14*, 81-90.

Weatherhead, A. D. Psychogenic headache. *Headache*, 1980, *20*, 47-54.

Whatmore, G. B., & Kohli, D. R. *The physiopathology and treatment of functional disorders.* New York: Grune & Stratton, 1974.

Wilkinson, M., & Woodrow, J. Migraine and weather. *Headache*, 1979, *19*, 375-378.

Wolff, H. G. Personality features and reactions of subjects with migraine. *Archives of Neurology and Psychiatry*, 1937, *37*, 895-921.

Yates, A. J. *Biofeedback and the modification of behavior.* New York: Plenum Press, 1980.

Ziegler, D. K. Genetics of migraine. *Headache*, 1977, *16*, 330-331.

Ziegler, D. K. Headache syndromes: Problems of definition. *Psychosomatics,* 1979, *20,* 443–447.

Ziegler, D. K., Hassanein, R. S., & Couch, J. R. Characteristics of life headache histories in a non-clinic population. *Neurology,* 1977, *27,* 265–269.

Ziegler, D. K., Hassanein, R. S., Harris, D., & Stewart, R. Headache in a non-clinic twin population. *Headache,* 1975, *13,* 213–218.

Ziegler, D. K., Hassanein, R. S., & Hassanein, K. Headache syndromes suggested by factor analysis of symptom variables in a headache prone population. *Journal of Chronic Diseases,* 1972, *25,* 353–363.

Ziegler, D. K., & Stewart, R. Failure of tyramine to induce migraine. *Neurology,* 1977, *27,* 725–726.

Zung, W. W. K. A self-rating depression scale. *Archives of General Psychiatry,* 1965, *12,* 63–70.

Index

Ad Hoc Committee on the Classification of Headache, 50-54
Adolescents, headache symptoms in, 65-69
Allan, W., 7
Amitriptyline chloride, 82-83
Anderson, C. D., 35
Anderson, J. A. D., 115-116
Andersson, P. G., 85
Andrasik, F., 11, 102-103
Andreychuk, T., 116
Ansel, E. L., 116-117
Antidepressants, 82-83
Anxiolytics, 82
APC and APC-like drugs, 81-82
Appenzeller, O., 43
Attention-diversion training, 138-141, 144
Autonomic epilepsy, 42
Autonomic nervous system, headaches and, 42-44, 72-76

Bakal, D. A., 12-13, 20, 34, 35, 43, 60-62, 63, 69, 71-76, 86, 94, 112-114
Barber, T. X., 116
Basmajian, J. V., 35
Beecher, H. K., 45-46, 88-89
Behavioral aproaches to headache treatment, 100, 118-119
  biofeedback, 100-109, 131-138
  cognitive skill training, 109-118, 138-147
Bibace, R., 17
Bille, B. O., 66-67
Biochemistry of headache, 27-47
Biofeedback training, 100-109, 131-138
Blanchard, E. B., 58-59
Budzynski, T. H., 101-102, 129

Cameron, R., 121-122
Catastrophizing cognitions, 16
Cerebral blood flow, 38-42
Children, headache symptoms in, 65-69
Chocolate, 94-95
Classic migraine, 50-52
Cluster headache, 51, 79
Cognition of headache, 16-18
  coping styles and, 18-26
Cognitive behavioral treatment program, 120-123
  attention-diversion training, 138-141
  imagery training, 141-145
  patient's conceptualization of headache, 123-126
  relaxation/biofeedback training, 126-138
  thought management, 145-147

161

Cognitive skills training, 109–118, 138–147
Cohen, F., 19–20
Cohen, M. J., 43, 105–107
Common migraine, 50–52
Conversion reaction headache, 51–52
Conversion V, 24
Coping with headache
  dispositional and process approaches, 19–21
  self-statements for, 145, 146–147
  susceptibility and, 18–26
Couch, J. R., 25, 82–83, 84
Coyne, J. C., 13–14
Curran, D. A., 47
Cylinder analogy, 1–3

Dalessio, D. J., 30, 32, 46, 83, 95
Dalsgaard-Nielsen, T., 11
Dalton, K., 98
Demjen, S., 22, 23
Depression headache, 25–26, 51–52
  antidepressants, 82–83
Description versus diagnosis, 80
Deubner, D. C., 65, 67
Diamond, S., 25, 50–52, 53, 58, 80
Diets and headaches, 97
Distress versus stress, 10–26
Doppler ophthalmic test, 32–33
Drugs
  in headache management, 81–92
  and headache-related behavior, 86–92
  for migraine, 83–86
  for muscle-contraction headache, 81–83
Duration of headache, 56–60

Edmeads, J., 29
EEG feedback, 101–102, 105
Elmore, A. M., 105, 106
EMG feedback, 31, 34–37, 101–103, 105, 111, 113, 133–134. See also Biofeedback training

Ergotamine tartrate, 84–86
Evans, F. J., 81, 89

Familial incidence of headache, 5–9
Fasting and headaches, 96–97
Foodstuffs and headaches, 94–96
Frank, R. T., 98
Frankl, V. E., 1–2
French, E. B., 43
Frequency of headaches, 53–54, 60–62, 123–126, 127. See also Symptoms
Friar, L. R., 104
Friedman, A. P., 56, 78

Gate-control theory, 45
General adaptation syndrome, x
General systems approach, 4–5
Genest, M., 45, 121, 139, 141
Genetic predisposition, 5–9
Goodell, H., 7
Graham, J. R., 6, 28

Hakkarainen, H., 85
Harding, H. C., 115, 116
Harper, R. G., 24–25
Headache
  classification of, 50–55
  conceptualization of, 123–126
  physical triggers of, 92–98
  see also Symptoms
Headache assessment questionnaire, 134, 135–137
Headache frequency record, 53–54, 60–62, 123–126, 127
Headache personality, 20
Headache treatment
  biofeedback training, 100–109, 131–138
  cognitive behavioral program, 120–150
  cognitive skills training, 109–118, 138–147
  drugs in, 81–92
Hemiplegic migraine, 50–51

Index

Henryk-Gutt, R., 11
Hereditary headache, 5-9
Hockaday, J. M., 43
Holistic approach, viii-ix, 3-4, 77, 81. *See also* Psychobiological model
Holroyd, K., 35, 111-112
Hunter, M., 58
Hypnosis, 115-118
Hypochondriasis, 20-25

Illness Behavior Questionnaire, 22-23
Imagery training, 141-145
Inflammatory headache, 51
Ingvar, D. H., 42
Intracranial blood flow, 38-42

Jay, G. W., 65
Jessup, B. A., 96, 102, 104-105
Joffe, R., 67-69

Kaganov, J. A., 71-76, 98
Kudrow, L., 23, 25, 32, 54
Kunkel, R. S., 60-62, 65, 78

Lance, J. W., 6, 54
Lazarus, R. S., 3-4, 13-14
Legewie, H., 107-108
Levendusky, P., 90-91
Lucas, R. N., 8

Marcusson, R. M., 11
Masked depression, 25
Mason, J. W., 96-97
Mathew, N. T., 40, 41
McGill Pain Questionnaire, 58
Medina, J. L., 97
Meichenbaum, D., 16, 109-110, 121
Melzack, R., 26, 45, 58
Menstrual migraine, 98-99
Migraine headache, ix-x
  autonomic instability and, 42-44
  classification of, 50-55
  drugs for, 83-86
  menstrual, 98-99

precipitants of, 92-98
psychosomatic, 21
vascular mechanisms and, 28-32
weekend, 15
see also Symptoms
Migraine–muscle-contraction headache dichotomy, 31, 48-50, 52-55, 80. *See also* Symptoms
Minnesota Multiphasic Personality Inventory, 24-25, 109
Moffett, A. M., 94
Monosodium glutamate, 94
Morley, S., 43
Muscle-contraction headache, ix-x
  classification of, 50-55
  drugs for, 81-83
  see also Symptoms
Musculoskeletal activity and headache, 33-38, 72-76

Nausea, 52-53, 56-60. *See also* Migraine headache; Symptoms

O'Brien, M. D., 39-40
Olesen, J., 37, 52-53, 59-60, 64, 84, 85-86
Onset of headache, 10-14, 54
Ophthalmoplegic migraine, 50-51
Otis, S. M., 32, 33

Pain, headache, 16-17, 44-47. *See also* Physiological mechanisms; Symptoms
Parnell, P., 86
Pearce, P., 21
Phenylethylamine, 94-95
Philips, C., 24, 34-35, 53, 58
Physical triggers of headaches, 92-98
Physiological mechanisms, 28-29
  autonomic nervous system, 42-44
  cerebral blood flow, 38-42
  musculoskeletal activity, 33-38
  pain, origin of, 44-47
  vascular mechanisms, 28-33
Pilowsky, I., 22-23

Placebos, 87–92
Population, headache symptoms of, 70–76
Pózniak-Patewicz, E., 34
Premenstrual syndrome, 98
Price, K. P., 44
Process-oriented approach, 14
Prodromal symptoms, 57, 79. *See also* Symptoms
Prophylactic drugs, 83–84
Psychobiological model, x, 1–9, 77–80, 92–98
Psychobiological predisposition, 5–9
Psychogenic headache, 22–23
Psychosomatic migraine, 21

Regional cerebral blood flow, 39–42
Relaxation training, 107–108, 113, 114, 116, 126–131
Ruble, D. N., 98–99

Sacks, O., 6–7, 9
Sakai, F., 40–41
Sargent, J. D., 101–102
Schwartz, G., 4
Self-observation headache records, 123–126, 127
Self-statements for coping with headache, 145, 146–147
Selye, H., x
Serotonin, 46–47
Severity model, x. *See also* Psychobiological model
Shapiro, A. K., 87–88, 89
Sicuteri, F., 46–47
Simard, D., 40
Skinhøj, E., 40
Smith, C. H., 43
Sovak, M., 104, 109
Spanos, N. P., 117–118
Specificity/generality assumption, 101–109
Sternbach, R. A., 3, 24
Stress versus distress, 10–26
Susceptibility to headache, 18–26, 33–38

Symptoms, 48–50
 in children, 65–69
 classification of headaches and, 50–55
 empirical observation of, 55–65
 in population, 70–76
Symptoms of psychopathology, 24

Temperature training, 101–109, 114, 116, 117
Tension headache, *see* Muscle-contraction headache
Tfelt-Hansen, P., 35
Thompson, J. K., 72
Thought management, 145–147
Thought versus cognition, 17–18
Throbbing pain, 56–60
Toxic vascular headache, 51
Traction headache, 51
Transaction, defined, 3–4
Tunis, M. M., 31
Turin, A., 103
Turk, D. C., 102, 103, 121, 143–144, 145, 146–147
Tursky, B., 58
Tyramine, 94–96

Ultrasonic transducers, 31–33
Unilateral pain, 56–60

Vascular mechanisms, 28–33, 72–76
Vascular migraine headache, 50–55
Vomiting, 52–53, 56–60. *See also* Migraine headache; Symptoms

Waters, W. E., 7–8, 70–71
Weather, migraines and, 93–94
Weekend migraine, 15
Whatmore, G. B., 18
Wilkinson, M., 93–94
Wolff, H. G., 10–11, 20, 28–31, 37–38, 49, 118–119

Yates, A. J., 101, 108–109

Ziegler, D. K., 7, 8, 55, 56–57, 71, 94–95
Zung, W. W. K., 25–26